KU-262-308

CONTENTS

Foreword ix
Preface xiii
Acknowledgments xv

PART I — The Need for Public–Private Partnerships in Physical Activity and Health

CHAPTER 1 **Finding Consensus in Developing Partnerships . . . 5**

Defining Partnerships 6
Role of Partnerships in Physical Activity and Health 14
Conclusion. 16

CHAPTER 2 *The Partnership Protocol* **. 17**

ParticipACTION 19
The Partnership Protocol 21
Guidelines for Effective Partnerships. 24
Conclusion. 26

PART II — Public–Private Partnership Strategies

CHAPTER 3 **Basics of Messaging and Marketing in Physical Activity and Health. 29**

Importance of a Good Communications Strategy 31
Communications Strategies 32
Marketing for Behavioral Change 37
Communicating Through Social Media. 41
Harnessing Tools of Inactivity to Promote Physical Activity 43
Communicating Across Cultures. 44
Conclusion. 49

CHAPTER 4   **The Value of Sponsorship in Physical Activity, Sport Participation, and Health** **51**

Image Transfer 53
Stakeholders: Sponsors, Sponsees, and Agencies 54
Size and Scope of the Sponsorship Industry 57
Strategic Sponsorship 57
Finding a Sponsor for Your Not-for-Profit 60
Profile of a Sponsee 65
Finding a Not-for-Profit Sponsee for Your For-Profit Corporation 66
Profile of a Sponsor 67
Conclusion. 67

CHAPTER 5   **Revenue Strategies for Not-for-Profit Organizations.** **69**

Data on Sport and Recreation Organizations 70
Government Sources 71
Fees for Goods and Services. 72
Philanthropic Sources. 73
Conclusion. 77

CHAPTER 6   **Dimensions of Corporate Philanthropy and Partnerships** **79**

Corporate Support for Not-for-Profits 80
Corporate Donations 84
In-Kind Donations of Goods and Services 88
Sponsorships 89
Cause-Related Marketing 90
Employee Volunteering. 91
Conclusion. 92

CHAPTER 7   **Role Models and Champions** **93**

Role Models. 94
From Role Model to Champion 98
Champions in Action 107
Conclusion. 112

CHAPTER 8   **Leveraging Corporate Social Responsibility to Partner With Corporations** **113**

Introducing CSR. 114
Corporate Perspective on Partnerships 115
Integrate CSR to Attract Partners 115

Public–Private Partnerships in Physical Activity and Sport

Physical Activity Intervention Series

Norm O'Reilly, PhD
Ottawa University

Michelle K. Brunette, MHK
Laurentian University

**Evidence-based guidelines for successful collaboration
from *The Partnership Protocol***

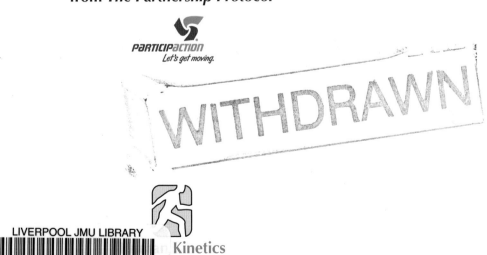

Kinetics

Library of Congress Cataloging-in-Publication Data

O'Reilly, Norm, 1973-
    Public-private partnerships in physical activity and sport / Norm O'Reilly and Michelle K. Brunette.
      p. ; cm. -- (Physical activity intervention series)
    Includes bibliographical references and index.
  I. Brunette, Michelle K., 1978- II. Title. III. Series: Physical activity intervention series.
    [DNLM: 1. Physical Fitness. 2. Exercise. 3. Health Promotion. 4. Public-Private Sector Partnerships.
    5. Sports. QT 255]

  613.7--dc23

2012031836

ISBN-10: 1-4504-2187-3 (print)
ISBN-13: 978-1-4504-2187-4 (print)

The web addresses cited in this text were current as of November 2012, unless otherwise noted.

Acquisitions Editor: Myles Schrag; **Developmental Editor:** Melissa J. Zavala; **Assistant Editors:** Amy Akin and Casey A. Gentis; **Copyeditor:** Bob Replinger; **Indexer:** Nancy Ball; **Permissions Manager:** Dalene Reeder; **Graphic Designer:** Nancy Rasmus; **Graphic Artist:** Yvonne Griffith; **Cover Designer:** Keith Blomberg; **Photograph (cover):** © Human Kinetics; **Photo Production Manager:** Jason Allen; **Art Manager:** Kelly Hendren; **Associate Art Manager:** Alan L. Wilborn; **Illustrations:** © Human Kinetics; **Printer:** Versa Press

Printed in the United States of America   10 9 8 7 6 5 4 3 2 1

The paper in this book is certified under a sustainable forestry program.

Human Kinetics
Website: www.HumanKinetics.com

United States: Human Kinetics
P.O. Box 5076
Champaign, IL 61825-5076
800-747-4457
e-mail: humank@hkusa.com

Canada: Human Kinetics
475 Devonshire Road Unit 100
Windsor, ON N8Y 2L5
800-465-7301 (in Canada only)
e-mail: info@hkcanada.com

Europe: Human Kinetics
107 Bradford Road
Stanningley
Leeds LS28 6AT, United Kingdom
+44 (0) 113 255 5665
e-mail: hk@hkeurope.com

Australia: Human Kinetics
57A Price Avenue
Lower Mitcham, South Australia 5062
08 8372 0999
e-mail: info@hkaustralia.com

New Zealand: Human Kinetics
P.O. Box 80
Torrens Park, South Australia 5062
0800 222 062
e-mail: info@hknewzealand.com

E5620

To our favorite partners, Nadège, Emma, Kian, Thomas, and Leland, and Jamie, Malin, and Nellie

How CSR Can Improve Partnerships 121
Examples of CSR in Partnerships 124
Conclusion 130

PART III **Putting Partnership Guidelines Into Action**

CHAPTER 9 **Global, National, and Community Partnership Perspectives** **133**

Partnering Across Sectors 134
Global Perspectives 135
Conclusion 151

CHAPTER 10 **Applying Partnership Guidelines in Physical Activity and Health** **153**

CATCH Case Study 154
Partnership Examples 164
Conclusion 165

CHAPTER 11 **Challenges in Creating Effective Partnerships: Bias, Controversy, and Failure** **169**

Measuring Partnership Effectiveness 170
Elements of an Effective Partnership 171
Key Partnership Challenges 175
Avoiding Partnership Breakdown Through Good Management 181
Conclusion 182

Appendix A   The Science Behind Developing
The Partnership Protocol 185
Appendix B   *The Partnership Protocol* 189
Epilogue 205
Glossary 209
References 213
Index 223
About the Authors 231

FOREWORD

It is with distinct pleasure that I write the foreword to this book. I believe strongly in the concept of partnerships with the private sector by the not-for-profit sector.

Partnerships between not-for-profit organizations in the sport, health, and physical activity realms (and beyond) and the private sector have attracted the interest of media and academia, as well as those in industry. In my view, these partnerships become even more relevant as we move further into the 21st century, given the scarcity of resources and increasing competition for government support and funding.

My perspective is uncommon in that I have devoted my professional career to working in both the for-profit and not-for-profit worlds. Perhaps that is the reason that I value these partnerships so highly and know that they can be effective. I left the private sector for the not-for-profit sector because I would like to contribute to changing the world. I believe that it is possible to change the world if, and only if, the public, private, and not-for-profit sectors work together, arm in arm. We must change the world. We can change the world. Through effective and responsible partnerships between the three sectors, we will change the world.

When I was invited to write the foreword to this book, I eagerly accepted the offer. I take great pride in this book being published because it is one of the many outputs that resulted from the efforts of a working group that my organization, ParticipACTION, initiated during the summer of 2009. At the time, this group embarked on a project, *The Partnership Protocol*, to improve, support, and facilitate more and better partnerships in our sector, related sectors, and, in reality, any sector. At that time, we created a steering committee to drive the project. I assumed the role of committee chair, and Dr. O'Reilly assumed the role of committee secretariat. The committee was composed of leaders from diverse backgrounds, including a beverage manufacturer, a food manufacturer, universities, a marketing agency, and not-for-profit organizations. This group had a mandate to research, discuss, and incubate the creation of guidelines for successful public–private partnerships. Their specific objective was to develop guidelines that would assist not-for-profits, of all shapes and sizes, in the fields of sport and physical activity to find, implement, and sustain responsible, effective partnerships with the private sector.

An important aspect of the committee's work, and one that is emphasized in this book, is the focus on sustainable and responsible partnerships. By sustainable, I mean long term, in which the efforts simultaneously support the respective goals of all organizations involved in the partnership. By responsible, I refer to the requirement that these partnerships are responsible to the external groups affected, including the general population.

Throughout the 18-month effort of the steering committee, we embarked on a collaborative process that was based on a strong foundation of research and obtained input from key stakeholders. This vitally important approach is captured and described in this book.

Whether you are from the for-profit or not-for-profit sector, or even if you are a boundary spanner who works in both, I encourage you to use the research, concepts, ideas, and tactics presented in this book to expand and improve your partnership activities. I am confident that by working together, arm in arm, in highly effective partnerships across all sectors, we really will change the world for ourselves, for our children, for the better!

Enthusiastically,

Kelly D. Murumets
President and CEO, ParticipACTION
Chair, *The Partnership Protocol* Steering Committee

Bio

Photo courtesy of Kelly Murumets.

Kelly is the president and CEO of ParticipACTION, the national voice of physical activity and sport participation in Canada. ParticipACTION has been an iconic Canadian brand since 1971 and was relaunched under Kelly's dynamic leadership in 2007.

Kelly is a passionate leader who has a history of effecting change in organizations. Before joining ParticipACTION, she was president of a publicly traded U.S. telecommunications company, where she oversaw the integration of four bankrupt or nearly bankrupt companies into one thriving organization that ranked seventh in Deloitte's Technology Fast 50 Program. Kelly is a member of the Young Presidents' Organization (YPO) and has advised leaders from Canada, the United States, South America, and Europe on how to develop focused strategies and realize results within their organizations.

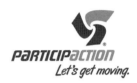

Reprinted, by permission, from ParticipACTION.

Kelly has been involved with the not-for-profit sector throughout her career. She is a member of the Bishop's University Board of Governors, a member of the Dean's Advisory Council for the Laurier School of Business and Economics, and a director of ParticipACTION. She has worked and volunteered for the Children's Aid Society and Covenant House and speaks regularly to organizations across the country.

She holds an MBA from the Richard Ivey School of Business at the University of Western Ontario, a master's of social work from Wilfrid Laurier University (WLU), and a BA from Bishop's University. Kelly won the Governor General's Academic Medal and the Gold Medal at WLU and is a member of the Golden Key International Honour Society.

Kelly was named to the 2007 and 2009 Canadian Association for the Advancement of Women and Sport and Physical Activity (CAAWS) Most Influential Women in Sport and Physical Activity list, named an Amazing Advocate on *More Magazine*'s Top 40 over 40 list for 2009, and recently was named to Canada's Most Powerful Women: Top 100.

Kelly brings her passion for sport and physical activity to her personal pursuits. She enjoys skiing and scuba diving and has climbed Mount Kilimanjaro and Mount Rainier.

PREFACE

In the true spirit of partnership, this book comes from the collaboration of many minds. Indeed, the first steps on the path that led to this book were inspired by a group of leaders who identified the need to formalize, conceptualize, and provide direction on partnerships between the public sector and the private sector. This collaborative process and a focus on obtaining a variety of viewpoints from many stakeholders are fundamental to this book and are evident throughout.

Leaders from public and private organizations, athletes, and academics have contributed their perspectives to help shape the book and provide the reader with real and relevant examples of public–private partnerships in action. In almost every chapter, you will find Executive Perspectives in which leaders share their real-world partnership experiences and threads of advice that may help your organization succeed or grow in your partnership building. The leaders share important insider views and lessons learned about how to drive partnerships through quality, credibility, motivation, and mutual respect; how to communicate your message and market health with consistent messages and through the tools of social media; how to reach youth and multicultural target groups; how to use philanthropy and corporate social responsibility; and how to be true to your organization's values and priorities. Following each Executive Perspective, a series of Global Application Questions are aimed at helping you contextualize the perspective and chapter, especially in relation to your organization and your goals and objectives. Through the chapters, a few interesting Partnership Highlights are presented as real-world case studies of partnerships in action (see chapter 4 for an example of how partners come together for parkland rejuvenation, and see chapter 9 for Nike's long reach in global, national, and local partnership building). The book is designed as a guide for not-for-profit, charity, and sport organizations to develop and maintain partnerships with corporate and government partners. It emphasizes how to make a partnership work most effectively for the reader's organization and within its resources, scope, and purpose. Similarly, the content of the book is highly relevant to private-sector corporations seeking to partner with the public sector and to agencies seeking to broker such partnerships.

eBook
available at
HumanKinetics.com

Because partnerships are growing realities for health, sport, and physical activity organizations and because these organizations are providing a growing medium for corporate-sector partners to meet their objectives, the content of this book provides background for university and college students in the fields of business, sports administration, physical education, health promotion, political science, and community development, as well as for practitioners in these fields.

ACKNOWLEDGMENTS

Special thanks to chapter 5 and 6 guest coauthor Steven Ayer, President, Common Good Strategies

Elio Antunes, COO and VP of Partnerships, ParticipACTION

Tammy Belanger, Race Participant, Sudbury ROCKS!!! Race Run Walk for Diabetes

John-Paul Cody-Cox, Chief Executive Officer, Speed Skating Canada

Kevin Compton, Managing Partner, Radar Partners and Majority Owner, Silicon Valley Sports and Entertainment

Bev Deeth, President and CEO, Concerned Children's Advertisers (CCA)

Annie Gregoire, Chef de groupe, Garnier Coloration

Chuck Hamilton, Social Learning Leader, IBM Center for Advanced Learning

Mark Harrison, President, TrojanOne

Eric Hentges, Executive Director, International Life Sciences Institute (ILSI) North America

Peter Katzmarzyk, Associate Executive Director for Population Science, Pennington Biomedical Research Center

Becky Lankenau, Director of the Centers for Disease Control and Prevention (CDC)–World Health Organization (WHO) Collaborating Center for Physical Activity and Health

Craig Larsen, Executive Director, Chronic Disease Prevention Alliance of Canada

Aaron Logan, President, Heritage Stick Company

Don Lord, Researcher, Nipissing University, University of Ottawa

Christine Lowry, Vice President, International Nutrition, Kellogg Company, Vice President, Nutrition and Corporate Affairs, Kellogg Canada Inc.

Steve Lusk, Consultant, FlagHouse

Lauren K. MacDonald, Marketing Manager, Gatorade at PepsiCo Canada

Jennifer MacKinnon, Regional Director (North East Ontario), Canadian Diabetes Association

Camon Mak, Director, Newcomer and Multicultural Markets, RBC Royal Bank of Canada

Paul Melia, President and CEO, Canadian Centre for Ethics in Sport and Chair of the Board, True Sport

Dave Moran, Director of Sustainability and Community Investment, Coca-Cola Canada

Kelly D. Murumets, President and CEO, ParticipACTION

Vince Perdue, President, Sudbury ROCKS!!! Running Club, Race Director, Sudbury ROCKS!!! Race Run Walk for Diabetes

Chris Pirie, Researcher at the Institute for Sport Marketing (ISM), Laurentian University

Richard Pound, International Olympic Committee

Julia Porter, Deputy Director, Education and Aboriginal Initiatives, Right To Play Canada

Elia Saikaly, Founder, FindingLife and FindingLife Films

Art Salmon, Team Leader: Research, Ontario Ministry of Health Promotion

Scott Smith, Chief Operating Officer, Hockey Canada

Mark Tremblay, Director, Healthy Active Living and Obesity Research Group, Children's Hospital of Eastern Ontario Research Institute

Anne Warner, JumpStart

The authors also wish to express a special thanks to the reviewers and publishing team at Human Kinetics.

The Need for Public–Private Partnerships in Physical Activity and Health

Our work over the past few years has led us across North America in search of information, data, and input on partnerships between the private sector and the public sector. We have heard from those who believe passionately in these partnerships and from those who are diametrically opposed to these partnerships, as well as many who fall somewhere in between. Our observation from these consultations with hundreds of industry experts and thousands of pages of related research, publications, and data in the area is that, although both views (pro and con) are valid, most in the industry views these partnerships as a needed source or revenue for not-for-profit sport, health, and physical activity organizations. This need, based on our observations, is supported by five important facts.

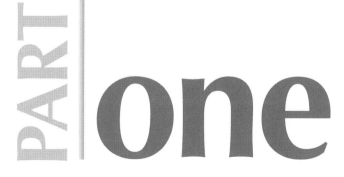

PART one

1

First, from reviewing research in a variety of sectors, we know that partnerships are a key element of any successful organization (see Trafford and Proctor 2006). Partnerships, when done properly, expand markets, increase efficiency, provide resources, allow access to expertise, and provide platforms for marketing, activation, and programs.

Second, an inactivity crisis is occurring in many developed countries, where both adult and youth activity levels have been decreasing for many years (see Colley et al. 2011). This development has implications for health care (increasing costs, lifestyle-related medical problems, and so on), sport, and physical activity (role in improving health behaviors).

Third, because of an increasing number of not-for-profit organizations in the areas of health, sport, and physical activity, as well as the increasing costs to governments of core health care and education, resources are becoming increasingly scarce for not-for-profit organizations in these sectors (Foster et al. 2009). These trends, in turn, create increased competition for existing public-sector financial resources (e.g., government, foundations, and not-for-profits) and nonfinancial resources (e.g., volunteers, in-kind donations of services or products), leading public-sector organizations to seek alternative sources of funding, including partnerships with the private sector (Babiak and Thibault 2009).

Fourth, on the other side of these partnerships, we have observed that private-sector organizations are increasingly interested in not-for-profit physical activity, health, and sport partners. Corporations have recognized that these not-for-profit partners can provide the corporate partner with valuable links to potential markets and brand associations that are not easily obtained from other sources. The rationale for this is based on sponsorship research (for a copy of the Sixth Annual Canadian Sponsorship Landscape Study, visit www.sponsorshiplandscape.ca), which notes that (a) a large proportion of sponsorship resources are invested in not-for-profit properties (a.k.a., sponsees); (b) the mix of properties that sponsors invest in is becoming increasingly diverse and less dominated by professional sport; and (c) industry experts have identified, year over year for the five years of the landscape study, increased activation, more use of social media, and improved evaluation and servicing more in line with sponsor needs. These findings can be extrapolated further, supporting our position.

Fifth, and finally (and perhaps most important), the controversy related to partnerships that not-for-profit health, sport, and physical activity properties enter into with the private sector would benefit from being addressed. The controversy arises when the not-for-profit partner enters into a partnership with a private-sector partner who has objectives that differ considerably from those of the not-for-profit partner (e.g., a beverage company and a medical association). Although this gap in objectives is what allows the not-for-profit partner to accrue considerable revenues and enable other revenue-generating activities, it simultaneously draws negative media interest, which, perhaps counterintuitively, is largely and commonly directed at the sponsee partner, not the corporate partner. The rationale for raising this issue is that more responsible and effective implementation of these partnerships will benefit all parties involved.

Given the context, industry interest, and supported rationale laid out, we believe that the need for this book and its content is strongly justified.

CHAPTER 1

Finding Consensus
in Developing Partnerships

One of the predictors of reaching a health goal is sharing your goals with a partner. It may be in the form of a workout partner ready to set fitness challenges with you, a commitment that you make to be part of a sport team, or an online community of people sharing their fitness targets. Just like individuals who establish health goals, physical activity, sport, and health organizations may find success in meeting their desired targets and objectives by partnering with other organizations. Partnerships work. Partnerships provide benefits to both partners.

Partnerships take multiple forms and have numerous purposes, but in many cases partnering can bring each partner a myriad of benefits. In this chapter we examine partnership structures across various public and private sectors. We consider how different strengths of partnering and commitments are related to the partnership's purposes and outcomes, especially to the role of partnerships in promoting physical activity, sport participation, and health. In times when obesity rates are skyrocketing across the globe and sport participation is declining, partnering offers organizations new ways to increase their profile and reach new members.

Because participation in sport and physical activity is decreasing or stagnating in communities (Vail 2007) and youth (Tremblay et al. 2010), sport organizations and community leaders must seek new ways to promote wellness, fitness, and healthy lifestyles. Because of the current global inactivity crisis and scarcity of resources, public (not-for-profit) organizations in the sport and physical activity context require guidance for successful and responsible partnering with private (for-profit) organizations. Advocates of sport participation, health promotion, and physical activity around the globe must become more strategic and innovative in their efforts to engage the private sector in the pursuit of their mission and search for the necessary resources in an ever-competitive and results-oriented environment. Partnering can allow organizations to increase their profile and gain new avenues to reach members. Considerable evidence supports the benefits of partnerships between public and private organizations, but there is a lack of consensus about what exactly constitutes a partnership. Linkages that are termed *partnerships* between public and private sectors exist in multiple forms that vary by goals, strength of ties, power balances, and financial and time commitments (Babiak and Thibault 2009; Barr 2007; Cousens et al. 2006; Hodge and Greve 2007; Weiermair, Peters, and Frehse 2008; Widdus 2001). Despite the breadth of the partnership concept, partnering has been a useful tool for health, sport, and physical activity advocates to help build, implement, and manage programs to increase participation rates and attempt to reverse overall health declines.

Defining Partnerships

Broadly, the term *partnership* describes a relationship between organizations. Partnerships vary widely, based on the kind of actors in the partnership, the partnership goals and strengths, and the nature of the financial contributions involved. Partnerships can be formed in multiple ways between two or more businesses, charities, sport organizations, community groups, local government offices, and other forms of organizations. Partnerships can be in the form of donations and philanthropic linkages, sponsorship agreements, or more collaborative partnerships in which each partner contributes to the development of a common goal or program. Partnerships vary in the strength of the partnership (i.e., commitment and longevity of the partnership) and the level of influence on the other partner's goals, objectives, and actions.

What Are Public–Private Partnerships?

In the various layers of partnerships, an emerging trend has been the partnering of not-for-profit and charity organizations with corporate businesses. The growth of partnerships between public and private organizations has responded to the growing challenges that public organizations face in terms of funding, competition, recognition, and participation. The public sector embraces diverse groups including not-for-profit organizations (i.e., charities, youth summer camps, universities, and so on), government departments, and nongovernmental organizations (NGOs). A public–private partnership (PPP) is a strategic initiative amongst two parties in which (a) the public partner refers to a not-for-profit sport or physical activity organization (e.g., KidsHealth, United States Triathlon Association, Hockey Canada), a multisport organization (e.g., United States Olympic Committee, Commonwealth Games Canada, World Anti-Doping Agency), a health organization involved in physical activity (e.g., World Health Organization), or a government department (e.g., Health Canada and Sport Canada, which are branches of the Canadian government responsible for health and sport, respectively, in Canada) that funds sport or physical activity organizations, and (b) the private partner refers to for-profit, generally corporate organizations, who operate independently of government and whose goals are based on providing return to shareholders, typically through revenue generation or brand enhancement. The private partner organizations include business retailers, manufacturers, service providers, professional sport teams, and media.

On the public side, partners can involve a range of areas, organizations, or causes that include sport and physical activity but also areas (sometimes related) such as facilities, health, education, entertainment, charities, national issues, environment, and diversity. Examples of public partners involved in partnerships with private organizations are numerous, including ParticipACTION, Right To Play, Government of Canada, City of Vancouver, National Cancer Institute, the U.S. President's Council on Fitness, Sports and Nutrition, and USA Track & Field. Public organizations may seek private partners for one or more reasons including (a) cash or in-kind products to make up for the scarce resources typically available; (b) the proliferation of causes seeking those resources; (c) the fact that government resources are increasingly focused on health and education; (d) the expertise that the private partner provides that the public organization rarely has; and (e) access to the customers, employees, communications platforms, and distribution channels of the private partner.

To private organizations, partnering with a public group can provide (a) brand equity, (b) legitimacy (i.e., association to a cause), (c) cash or in-kind products or services, (d) a physical facility, or (e) a tax benefit for the financial commitment to the partnership. In the private sphere, Nike, Coca-Cola, CIBC, Scotiabank, Barclays, and many others have played significant roles in partnerships related to sport and physical activity. The permutations and combinations of public–private partnerships that exist are vast.

Why Partnerships?

In general, partnerships allow two or more partners to share resources, expertise, and markets for mutually beneficial (but not always equal) outcomes. A public–private partnership involves at least one public organization and at least one private organization, each bringing assets to the table and contributing to the others' expressed goals and objectives. The private partner typically provides cash or in-kind products or services to the partnership in return for the benefits accrued for supporting something attached to a cause (brand, employee morale, giving back, long-term sales, and so on). The public partner typically receives resources (cash or in-kind) and provides a platform, linked to a cause, from which other partners can leverage. As Hersey et al. (2012) described, "Collaboration helps to build program and partner capacity" (p. 223).

Partnerships between public and private organizations encompass broad purposes. The City of Ottawa partnered with Thunderbird Management to create the Ottawa Superdome Sports Centre for multiple sports usage. ParticipACTION partnered with Coca-Cola to create a national active youth program, and a Hockey Canada partnership with Esso Canada introduced thousands of girls to hockey through free ice time and training programs. Even relatively small funding arrangements (so-called micro-philanthropy partnerships) can have big benefits for local community sport organizations. As Lornic (2010) noted, although public policy may not always encourage small-scale funding partnerships, the reality is that local projects are well suited to deliver "bang for the buck" by offering potential for better access and operation by people in the local community.

Partnerships Across Sectors

Organizations can benefit from engaging in partnerships with multiple sectors: (a) the health sector, (b) the sport sector, (c) the education sector, (d) the media, (e) local governments, and finally (f) national financial and economic policy makers, especially when the goal of the partnership is to promote physical activity (Right To Play 2008a). Accordingly, the health sector can provide evidence to advocate, inform, and build integrated networks with the public and policy makers of the health, social, and economic benefits of and barriers to physical activity. The sport sector can facilitate the use of sport facilities, allocate funds, provide sport training, and promote physical activities to all people regardless of ethnicity, social class, gender, or disability. The education sector can make school space available for community physical activity; commit to physical activity in the school curriculum; and encourage universities and colleges to undertake data collection, research, evaluation, and training for strategies to increase physical activity and set physical activity and sport as a platform for public education and communication. Schools are also prime sites for the delivery of physical activity and sport programs aimed at school-age children, teachers, and coaches (Right To Play 2008c). The media can promote physical activity through programming and positive messages and by educating their journalists to be advocates for physical activity. Local governments can support legislation and policies that promote safe and accessible indoor and outdoor physical activity spaces and programs. Finally, national financial and economic policy makers can allocate resources and encourage investment from the public and private sectors to support physical activity, sport, and other health promotion programs.

Partnership Continuum

Visualizing a partnership on a continuum can help capture the breadth of the term. On one end of the continuum would be partnerships with little influence on each other's actions. Each partner would independently determine goals and objectives, yet a partnership could exist by way of donations and other philanthropic linkages. On the other end of the continuum we could consider stronger partnerships, usually engaged in collaborative and cocreative activities. This end of this continuum, conceptually, would be the ideal partnership in which both organizations are contributing, activating, supporting the other's pursuit of its objectives, and so on. Within the sport and physical activity contexts, academic literature and corporate documents apply the term *partnership* to a variety of linkage models including (*a*) philanthropic linkages, (*b*) sponsorship linkages, and (*c*) collaborative partnerships (see figure 1.1). The motivation behind involvement is different for each type and can help us understand various relationships in sport and physical activity.

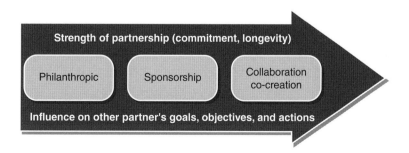

FIGURE 1.1 The partnership continuum.

Philanthropy

Philanthropic linkages refer to donations of money, time, or goods from a private enterprise to a public (usually charitable) organization or event. As with sponsorship agreements, the private donor is rarely included in setting the public organization's goals, visions, and practices. Often, donations can be on a yearly basis or dedicated for specific organization events. Donations may be made in response to either a crisis or a specific request. For example, the Mike Weir Foundation partnership with the RBC Canadian Open pro-am golf event exemplifies a donation-type linkage in which proceeds go to various children's health and wellness charities (Weir 2009). The private sphere may engage in philanthropic linkages to enhance the organization's community profile, gain access to new markets, increase corporate image, or generate good public relations (Widdus 2001). The motivation for engaging in these relationships is to build the reputation of the company as a good corporate citizen and to enhance brand loyalty. Donor companies engage in philanthropy either under duress to protect their reputation, to support projects of senior executives or board members, or to respond to a community crisis. Sport-related charities receive a large amount of individual donations compared with other causes. Many of the donations have little or no influence on the charity and represent informal giving commitments. But Steven Ayer, expert in not-for-profit marketing and former senior researcher at Imagine Canada, reminds us that the partnership continuum is not absolute in describing donor–sport charity relationships; some sport-related charities engage in philanthropic partnerships that are strong, long-term commitments built on a donor's sincere loyalty and belief in the sport organization's cause and values (Ayer 2011).

Sponsorship

In sponsorship relationships and linkages, the private organization acts as a financial donor or offers goods or services to the public organization, but the private organization has little input in establishing the goals and objectives of the public organization. Sponsorship linkages can provide financial contribution to a community or to large-scale sporting events (e.g., Canada Games), or provide funds, products, or services to national, provincial, or local sport organizations. Sponsor companies often feel pressure to form relationships because of the link between social responsibility and corporate success. This pressure comes from multiple sources, including an increase in requests from not-for-profits; government expectations of corporate contribution to society; and employee, customer, and shareholder expectations about corporate citizenship.

Notably, sponsorship resides in the middle of the continuum, often with stronger or more formal ties (e.g., sponsorship contracts) yet relatively low influence on the receiving partner's actions. For example, Hockey Canada's partnership list illustrates the broad conceptualization of the term *partnership*; partners are classified as premier (e.g., Esso), international (e.g., Air Canada), national (e.g., Egg Farmers of Canada), licensing (e.g., Old Time Hockey), or supplier partners (e.g., Easton) (Hockey Canada 2009). Despite the diverse types and strengths of relationships between the private organizations and Hockey Canada, the partnering is generally in the form of sponsorship agreements focused on financial contribution or exchanges of goods or services rather than direct influence by the private organizations on Hockey Canada's goals and visions.

Collaboration

Collaboration partnerships involve collaboration of efforts and input, usually in the form of a longer-term commitment, from both the public and the private sphere resulting in the cocreation of mutually beneficial outcomes (Hodge and Greve 2007; Weiermair, Peters, and Frehse 2008). In this regard, Cousens et al. (2006) noted that a true (collaborative) partnership implies that a high level of integration between partners is in place that includes formalized commitment to shared goals and visions. Partner organization may accept collective responsibility to improve society by leveraging their organization's key competencies and resources to contribute to broad, positive social outcomes. Partners often choose causes that are not directly linked with their own goods or services; rather, they address broad social issues that have far-reaching implications for society as a whole.

The benefits of a collaborative partnership are multiple. Partnerships between public and private organizations, as Hodge and Greve (2007) detailed, can allow the pooling of resources and the provision of ameliorated value for money in meeting the objectives of the partnership. Partnerships can share human, financial, and structural resources such as employees, financial capital, land, and equipment (Cousens et al. 2006). Public–private partnerships can improve the quality and speed of delivery of projects (Joyner 2007), gain specialized management and technology expertise (Pagdadis et al. 2008), increase productivity and professionalism (Weiermair, Peters, and Frehse 2008), and pull interest from new markets while pushing for more effective solutions to problems (Widdus 2001). As imperative as shared benefits, shared risk is identified in the literature as a basic tenet of a partnership (Barr 2007; Hodge and Greve 2007; Joyner 2007; Vining and Boardman 2008). Successful partnerships are efficient, predictable, and dependable in the way that resources are shared, the manner in which the partnership is managed, and in the delivery of the goals of the partnership (Babiak 2007).

Driving Partnerships
With Quality and Credibility

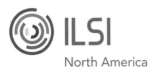

North America

Eric Hentges, PhD

Executive Director, International Life Sciences Institute
(ILSI) North America

BIO

Dr. Eric Hentges joined the International Life Sciences Institute, North America (ILSI NA) as the executive director in 2007. ILSI NA is a not-for-profit organization located in Washington, D.C., that provides a forum for academic, government, and industry scientists to identify and resolve nutrition and food safety issues important to the health of the public. Before taking this appointment Hentges served as the executive director of the U.S. Department of Agriculture Center for Nutrition Policy and Promotion. In this position he had oversight of the USDA's involvement in the development of the 2005 *Dietary Guidelines for Americans* and *MyPyramid, Food Guidance System*. Dr. Hentges has over 25 years of experience directing nutrition research, priority planning, and administration of competitive research grant programs for several national organizations. Additionally, he has led the development and implementation of nutrition education programs and consumer market research programs. Dr. Hentges holds degrees from Iowa State University, Auburn University, and Oklahoma State University. He is a member of the American Society for Nutrition and the Institute of Food Technologists.

VALUE OF PARTNERSHIPS

I am a firm believer in partnerships. Through partnering, organizations can benefit from increased audiences, shared resources, and increased trust and credibility. Each partner brings its own segment audience, so by partnering, organizations can more readily spread information and results to wider audiences. In times when resources are precious, partners can pool their resources, avoid wasting valuable time and effort, and build from one another rather than unnecessarily duplicate effort in reinventing the wheel. Partnerships are also able to increase trust and credibility because as more people come together, perceived trust in the issue increases. Specifically in partner-driven research, the assumption is that each member of the partnership has vetted and agreed on the issues presented, driving greater credibility in the results. The more viewpoints that are added to an issue, the less likely it is that an important point or perspective would be missed, avoiding segmentation.

CONSENSUS CONFERENCE ON OBESITY

Obesity is running rampant in North America, resulting in both an obesity epidemic and an epidemic of obesity programs. ILSI North America (NA) did not have its own research agenda related to obesity, but ILSI NA was interested in the science behind energy balance (energy in and energy out), which is critical to obesity programming. Following ILSI NA's partnership model of bringing together government, academia, and industry, a partnership was established with two top professional groups, the American Society for Nutrition and the American College of Sports Medicine, to develop a consensus conference on the role of energy balance in health and wellness. The aim of the conference is to bring to bear the best science to inform public policy directed toward the important obesity issue. Owing to the strength in the partnership, the conference results will be widely distributed in physical activity journals, nutrition journals, and presentations at several related conferences. They have the potential to encourage government groups to convene a national conference to deliver the results to targeted audiences and train-the-trainer events.

RISING ABOVE THE CRITICS

Even good coalitions can receive negative attention from groups who do not agree with the partnership's goals, objectives, or outcomes, or from people who believe that their needs were not being accurately represented. Strong support derived through partners, however, offers huge potential in overcoming the critics by adding credibility and quality and allowing the partnership to move forward.

DRIVING PARTNERSHIPS

Many United States government agencies have formal systems that encourage public–private partnerships in research. Regulatory bodies like the Food and Drug Administration (FDA) require industry to complete rigorous research before the FDA grants approval for new products. In this sense, the FDA's regulations advocate industry partnerships with research organizations in the process of expanding their markets through new product approval.

GLOBAL APPLICATION QUESTIONS

1. Dr. Hentges speaks to the importance of the global effects of the obesity crisis. How can international organizations use partnerships to further international efforts to reduce obesity?
2. Dr. Hentges emphasizes the ability of partnerships to expand communications beyond the ability of either individual partner. Provide three global examples of partnerships in which you believe this to be the case.
3. What are the benefits of partner-driven research?

SECOND HARVEST

The end goal of good research is typically publication in peer-reviewed literature. Dr. Hentges asks the question, "Then what?" The aim of a "second harvest" is to take results and get them out in the world, to put the results in action through multiple thought-leader groups at the state and county levels. By involving Nutrition Extension Programs in the second harvest of the Consensus Conference, the partnership will gain extension expertise that could more widely deliver the results in every state and

(continued) ▶

(continued) ▶

in universities. Drawing on an example, Dr. Hentges pointed to emerging science that linked heavy uses of low-calorie sweeteners with higher BMI. ILSI NA provided sound research identifying the cascade of responses from sweet-receptor stimulation, and the partnership with extension agents and educators can provide the second harvest by delivering information about the low-calorie sweetener and BMI relationship in a useable and timely way to local health and community organizations.

Role of Partnerships in Physical Activity and Health

The United Nations Inter-Agency Taskforce on Sport for Development and Peace defines sport broadly, including "all forms of physical activity that contribute to physical fitness, mental well-being and social interaction. These include: play; recreation; organized, casual or competitive sport; and indigenous sports or games" (Sport and Development 2009a). Sport and physical activity can generate health benefits through direct participation in the activity itself (e.g., increased health, fitness, and self-esteem) and through the use of participation and spectatorship as a platform to strengthen communication and connections, promote healthy attitudes and behaviors, and encourage social mobilization for multiple purposes (Bloom et al. 2005; Tremblay et al. 2010; Right To Play 2008a). In developing regions sport can be a powerful method to achieve policy objectives and mobilize societies; in Zambia sport has been a tool to prevent HIV–AIDS (Lindsey and Banda 2011), and sport has been used to promote agendas for peace and stability in other regions (Sport and Development 2009b).

In the world of sport and physical activity, developing partnerships make sense as a way to pool scarce resources. Linkages with private business and corporations give public, not-for-profit, and charity organizations an opportunity to build or increase strategic initiatives to meet a wealth of social, economic, and political needs aimed at increasing health, fitness, and participation in physical activity and sport.

Inactivity Crisis

Despite the benefits of sport, the declining rates of sport and physical activity participation by male and females of all ages further heighten the need for partnering, particularly given the evidence that this decline in fitness may lead to increases in chronic disease, higher health care costs, and possible decreases of productivity (Tremblay et al. 2010). Most developed countries report an alarming rise in youth obesity rates combined with decreased sport participation rates (O'Reilly 2010). The fitness levels of Canadians 6 to 19 years of age have declined significantly over the past three decades (Tremblay et al. 2010), and the health and fitness of adults 20 to 69 years old has decreased as well (Shields et al. 2010). ParticipACTION further detailed the inactivity crisis, pointing to the decline in sport participation rates in Canadian youth aged 15 to 18 from 77 percent to 59 percent and the decline in Canadian adult participation from 45 percent to 28 percent between 1992 and 2005 (Statistics Canada 2010). ParticipACTION also noted that the host of chronic degenerative conditions and the occurrence of premature death added to the estimated $5.3 billion annual cost to the economy and the $2.1 billion burden on the health care system (Katzmarzyk and Janssen 2004). Reversing the inactivity crisis and making regular physical activity and sport participation part of Canadians' lives can reduce all-cause mortality rates by as much as 30 percent (Andersen et al. 2000). The inactivity crisis is centered on both youth and adults, and the consequences are dire.

Amid decreased sport participation rates and declines in health, many countries see governments decreasing their support for not-for-profit organizations and sport organizations. According to Andersen et al. (2000), the decrease in government support has generally stemmed from cutbacks in government spending on physical activity and sport and an increase in the proportion of tax dollars required for core health care and education services. Because Canada and other countries are also facing proposed tax restrictions on donations to amateur sport organizations (Waldie 2011), the need for partnerships is steadily growing. At the same time, governments are setting expectations that the organizations that they do support should generate additional funding from external partners.

Benefits of Partnerships Good for Physical Activity and Health

Consider the desire to increase active transportation strategies in municipalities, such as walking trails, bike paths, and hiking routes. Community groups such as running and biking clubs, environmental groups, and outdoor enthusiasts may come together to identify needs and appropriate uses of trails and modes of active transportation. They may then look to partnerships with local municipalities who may be able to recognize the value of active transportation options on the health of their citizens but may be limited in their ability to fund the projects. With support from municipalities, community groups may be able to identify business leaders and organizations that could provide financing and help achieve the vision through promotion and marketing support. In the end, such partnerships can create new opportunities for physical activity to promote health, providing benefits to all partners and their members.

Farag and Brittain (2009) noted that over the past two decades many municipalities have entered into partnerships to provide sport and recreation facilities for their communities. Most of these projects have involved the creation or extensive renovation of medium-scale facilities, which often host minor-league professional sport teams and community events, which in turn create new employment opportunities. In Canada over 260,000 jobs are directly attributed to the sport economy, and Canadian households spend an estimated $15.8 billion on sport (Berger et al. 2008). Municipalities usually use some form of public–private partnership for these projects to achieve the objectives of limiting the municipality's financial exposure, taking advantage of private-sector financial resources, and taking advantage of private-sector expertise in facility design, marketing, and facility operations.

Partnerships can enhance the image of each organizational partner because sport and physical activity is generally seen in a positive way. The advantages of cooperation are obvious according to Weiermair et al. (2008) because private businesses can gain from government-supported strategies to raise capital at lower cost and public institutions can profit from professional management in business plan developments, market expertise, human resource management, or simply business logistics.

Conclusion

There are many versions and visions of what constitutes a partnership, each with different strengths and commitments. Partnerships between public and private organizations can allow resources to be shared and strengths to be amplified. Whether philanthropic, sponsorship, or more collaborative in nature, partnering brings together expertise from other sectors and allows partners to build toward a shared goal or values. Partnerships can play an important role in physical activity and health, helping to address the growing rates of inactivity and accompanying dire health consequences.

Moving forward, your organization can consider ways to use marketing and social media to promote your goals and partnership objectives. The value of sponsorship and fund-raising will be explored as relevant to the specific needs of your own organization. You can consider whether using role models and champions fits within the scope of your partnership and how your organization can use the growing trend of corporate social responsibility to further your vision in physical activity and health at the global, national, or community level. To put the partnership guidelines into practice, you can examine models of effective partnerships across multiple sectors and consider how to move beyond challenge and failures. Throughout the book, you'll learn from the wisdom of experts in the field of sport, physical activity, and health who share the lessons that they discovered from their own experiences in developing, maintaining, and managing partnerships.

In chapter 2 we will explore *The Partnership Protocol*, a ParticipACTION initiative detailing principles related to the creation, implementation, management, and evaluation of public–private partnerships. In choosing a partner, your organization will have to think critically about how you will manage your own and your partner's needs, advantages, and disadvantages, balanced with the needs of community stakeholders. *The Partnership Protocol* can serve as a guideline for choosing and working effectively with partners in multiple sectors.

CHAPTER 2

The Partnership Protocol

A 10-year-old girl looks down at her skates, stick in hand, and steps out on the ice. This is her first year playing hockey after years of hearing her single mother tell her that the equipment and registration fees just didn't fit the family budget. This year, with the help of the Canadian Tire Jumpstart Program, the little girl and many others like her will get a chance to participate in sport and recreation opportunities in their hometowns. The girl is benefitting from one of ParticipACTION's many partnerships with corporate partners that aim to increase the health and fitness levels of youth and adults in Canada. Guiding the way for other public organizations to establish effective partnerships with private businesses, ParticipACTION developed *The Partnership Protocol*. Leaders in organizations, especially not-for-profit and charity organizations, can use *The Partnership Protocol* and other partnership-building guidelines to assess their goals and objectives to build, maintain, and evaluate their partnerships in action.

To develop strong partnerships, organizations need a clear understanding of why each partner wishes to engage in a partnership by examining their individual needs, challenges, strengths, and opportunities. Thorough examination and proper planning can help increase the likelihood of developing a successful partnership. ParticipACTION, an organization that promotes initiatives for health and active living in Canada, developed guiding principles for organizations to develop and maintain effective partnerships. The purpose of *The Partnership Protocol, Principles and Approach for Successful Private/Not-for-Profit Partnerships in Physical Activity and Sport*, as detailed by Murumets et al. (2010), "is to provide not-for-profit organizations with evidence-informed guidance and a recommended approach to establishing, building, managing and evaluation of effective partnerships with the private sector in the advancement of physical activity and sport" (p. 1). The authors wish to express sincere thanks to ParticipACTION for allowing the reprint of *The Partnership Protocol* (see appendix B). *The Protocol* was developed with the expertise, insight, and best practices shared by a diverse set of over 300 stakeholders, led by a steering committee including Elio Antunes (COO and VP of partnerships, ParticipACTION); Mark Harrison (president, TrojanOne); Dr. Peter Katzmarzyk (associate executive director for Population Science, Pennington Biomedical Research Center); Chris Lowry (vice president, Nutrition & Corporate Affairs, Kellogg); Paul Melia (president and CEO, Canadian Centre for Ethics in Sport); David Moran (director, Public Affairs and Communications, Coca-Cola Canada); Kelly Murumets (president and CEO, ParticipACTION); Dr. Norm O'Reilly (associate professor of sport business, University of Ottawa); Dr. Art Salmon (team leader, Ministry of Health Promotion, Government of Ontario); and Dr. Mark Tremblay (director, Healthy Active Living and Obesity Research, Children's Hospital of Eastern Ontario Research Institute). *The Protocol*, Murumets et al. (2010) elaborated, was built on mutual understanding of each partner's goals, collaboration in communication strategies, and prioritization of resources to develop, implement, and evaluate the partnership. Because of the complexity and time sensitivity needed for the creation, implementation, management, and evaluation of partnerships, many practitioners strongly support *The Partnership Protocol* (e.g., at the 2011 Canadian Obesity Summit in Montreal, 74 percent of participants from not-for-profit, government, and private sectors ranked their support for *The Protocol* as high or very high [Tremblay 2011]). Recognizing the challenges of developing and maintaining effective partnerships to promote sport and physical activity, ParticipACTION designed *The Partnership Protocol* based on input from academic, government, business, and not-for-profit experts around the globe (ParticipACTION 2010).

ParticipACTION

ParticipACTION mobilizes the support of multisector partners to increase the physical health of Canadians by encouraging people to participate in sport and physical activities. ParticipACTION does not deliver programs directly, but in its leadership role, ParticipACTION facilitates collaborative partnerships through communication (e.g., delivering consistent and unified health promotion messages), capacity building (e.g., supporting the development of healthy programs), and knowledge exchange (e.g., research and reporting to appropriate stakeholders) (ParticipACTION 2009). ParticipACTION's "Get Inspired. Get Moving" multimedia campaign combined television commercials featuring renowned Canadian athletes and an online corkboard wall where athletes and ordinary Canadians shared stories to inspire others to be more active. Through formal, coordinated, and collaborative partnerships with Active Healthy Kids Canada, Boys and Girls Clubs of Canada, Canadian Space Agency, Coca-Cola, GreenGym, Loblaw Companies, SportChek, Sun Life Financial, Wilson Sporting Goods, and others, ParticipACTION develops, expands, or sustains physical activity programs though financial support and engagement with other not-for-profit partners (ParticipACTION 2009). According to ParticipACTION (2009), their partnership includes several initiatives, such as those presented in the following sections.

Improve the Grade

Improve the Grade is a report to parents on how to increase physical activity levels of their children through fitness, fun, and family. An insert detailing the findings of Canada's *Report Card on Physical Activity for Children and Youth* and advertisements in 600,000 copies of the *Globe and Mail* and *La Presse* were coupled with web resources, online promotions, and radio advertisements to encourage parents to increase movement, which, the initiative touted, could bring better academic results. See the Active Healthy Kids Canada *Report Card on Physical Activity for Children and Youth* (2009) for more information.

Canadian Tire Jumpstart Program

With the support of Wilson Sporting Goods and the Boys and Girls Club, ParticipACTION-branded basketballs, soccer balls, and footballs were sold at Canadian Tire. Proceeds were devoted to helping children in financial need participate in sport and physical activity through the Jumpstart program.

Get Fit for Space With Dr. Bob Thirsk

Partnering with the Canadian Space Agency, ParticipACTION challenged Canadians to enter their fitness data on the Canadian Space Agency website to virtually travel the 340 kilometers to the International Space Station. Each participant received a ParticipACTION pedometer and a personal (virtual) tour of the space station by Dr. Thirsk on their arrival.

Sogo Active

ParticipACTION partnered with Coca-Cola Canada Ltd. to reverse the declining sport and physical activity participation and the increasing time that children and adolescents spend in front of a computer or television screen. Through the Sogo Active program, teens (aged 13 to 19) could create and track their physical activity goals and network with friends or find physical activity resources, organizations, facilities, and equipment in their local areas. According to ParticipACTION (2009), "between November 2008 and June 2009, over 1,000 Sogo Active participants were selected by Coca-Cola Canada Ltd. to carry the Olympic Flame in the Vancouver 2010 Olympic Torch Relay" (p. 28).

GreenGym Partnership

Through ParticipACTION grants and its partnership with GreenGym, municipalities, schools, local organizations, and businesses were encouraged to install easy-to-use and weather-resistant outdoor fitness equipment in public spaces. GreenGyms are free to use and offer a wide range of activities to suit all needs using a person's own body weight for resistance.

Inspire the Nation

ParticipACTION and Sun Life Financial's coordinated and extensive communication efforts used an Inspiration Booth Caravan to bring to life the message "Get Inspired. Get Moving." Visiting 31 communities for media outreach, distributing 30,000 pedometers, and recording motivational physical activity stories from ordinary Canadians were all part of the campaign. Local partners, including YMCAs and recreational and public health departments, helped build excitement for the program.

The Partnership Protocol

The Partnership Protocol provides principles to guide the implementation of effective partnerships. Although ParticipACTION's *Partnership Protocol* is broad based, the unique strengths, goals, and design of organizations will also influence how the recommendations can be put into practice.

> *The Partnership Protocol* doesn't aim to answer the question of what is right for your organization, but to give you tools and information to help your organization find the best solutions possible for your needs. In the process, *The Partnership Protocol* provides an opportunity to debate, discuss and learn from other groups' partnerships. The ultimate goal of *The Partnership Protocol* is to increase capacity in the physical activity and sport sector, helping more Canadians to be more physically active.

ParticipACTION's *Partnership Protocol* (see figure 2.1) addresses three areas. Section 1, Why Partnerships? addresses the increasing need for not-for-profit organizations to enter into partnerships. Section 2 is titled Guiding Principles for Partnerships. Section 3, Approach to Effective Partnerships, suggests how to put those principles into practice in your organization. See appendix B for a complete discussion of *The Partnership Protocol*.

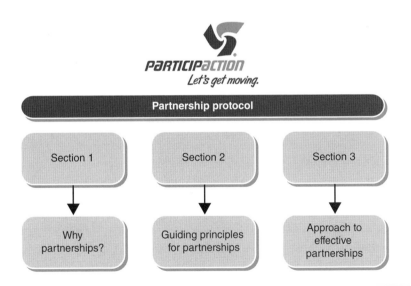

FIGURE 2.1   An overview of *The Partnership Protocol*.

Logo reprinted, by permission, from ParticipACTION.

Early Discussions and Motivation to Develop *The Partnership Protocol*

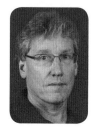

Mark Tremblay, PhD

Director, Healthy Active Living and Obesity Research Group,
Children's Hospital of Eastern Ontario Research Institute,
Ottawa, Ontario, Canada

BIO

Dr. Mark Tremblay has a bachelor of commerce degree in sports administration and a bachelor of physical and health education degree from Laurentian University. His graduate training was from the University of Toronto where he obtained his MSc and PhD from the Department of Community Health with a specialty in exercise science. Dr. Tremblay is the director of Healthy Active Living and Obesity Research (HALO) at the Children's Hospital of Eastern Ontario Research Institute and professor of pediatrics in the faculty of medicine, University of Ottawa, where he is also cross-appointed to the School of Human Kinetics and the Department of Epidemiology and Community Medicine. He is a fellow of the American College of Sports Medicine, chief scientific officer of Active Healthy Kids Canada, chair of the ParticipACTION Research Advisory Group, chair of the Canadian Physical Activity Guidelines Project, chair of the Canadian Health Measures Survey Expert Advisory Committee, and former dean of kinesiology at the University of Saskatchewan. Dr. Tremblay has published more than 130 papers and book chapters in the areas of childhood obesity, physical activity measurement, exercise physiology, exercise endocrinology, and health surveillance. He has delivered over 400 scholarly conference presentations, including more than 120 invited and keynote addresses, in 15 countries. Dr. Tremblay recently received an honorary doctorate from Nipissing University for his leadership contributions to healthy active living in Canada. Dr. Tremblay's most productive work has resulted from his 22-year marriage to his wife Helen, yielding four wonderful children.

BACKGROUND

With the arrival of the 21st century came the undeniable realization that an increased emphasis on health promotion and disease prevention was required for Canadians to preserve the quality of life to which they had become accustomed. Canadians of all ages were sitting more (Tremblay et al. 2010; Colley et al. 2011), moving less (Colley et al. 2011; Tremblay et al. 2008, 2005), and becoming less fit (Tremblay et al. 2010; Shields et al. 2010) and obese (Tremblay and Willms 2000; Tremblay et al. 2002; Shields et al. 2011) as a result. The estimated economic cost of our unhealthy lifestyle is unsustainable (Katzmarzyk and Janssen 2004), and it is predicted that our life expectancy will be reduced (Olshansky et al. 2005). The need for promotion, leadership, and advocacy for healthy active living has never been greater. Despite the obvious need, resources to support physical activity, sport, and active living organizations are scarce. And this problem was global.

FRUSTRATION AND MOTIVATION

As a board member of several national organizations involved in the promotion of healthy active living, I have become increasingly frustrated trying to operate with declining resources from both public and private sector sources in a climate of increased need and demand for services. Compounding this frustration was concern at the board table regarding who was an acceptable "partner." Occasionally a private-sector funding opportunity would present itself, but the organizational goals may be malaligned or there would be fear of retribution from sector partners who judged the partnership as inappropriate. Many hours, at various board tables, were spent agonizing over what constituted a good partnership and how to balance organizational needs and sector demands with perceived or real conflicts of interest or intentions. When projecting my personal experiences to the entire physical activity and sport sector, the toll of such debates on an already lean and stretched sector was substantial, repetitious, and inefficient.

Eventually, frustration led to motivation, and a small meeting with those experiencing similar frustrations was convened, initially just with representatives from Active Healthy Kids Canada (www.activehealthykids.ca) and ParticipACTION (www.ParticipACTION.com). At this meeting it was decided that it was a worthwhile endeavor to spend some time and resources to establish guiding principles for responsible partnerships in the physical activity and sport sector that would provide a roadmap for organizations to follow. These guidelines would provide not only a template for establishing responsible partnerships but also, if widely accepted and adopted, protection from the interorganizational judgments and conflicts resulting from externally perceived irresponsible partnerships.

PROCESS AND OUTCOME

ParticipACTION, the national voice for physical activity and sport in Canada, agreed to provide leadership for this initiative that would be developed and owned by the sector.

A multisectoral steering committee was formed with representatives from the physical activity and sport not-for-profit sector, private sector, government, and academia. The goal was to create a document, or set of guiding principles, or framework that would assist in the creation of public–private partnerships and reduce the cyclical debates occurring around volunteer board tables. A

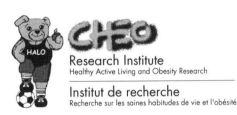

Reprinted, by permission, from CHEO Research Institute.

comprehensive search of relevant literature and an inclusive series of meetings and consultations were planned and carried out, and the product was *The Partnership Protocol,*

(continued) ▶

(continued) ▶

a guidebook for the assessment, development, implementation, management, and evaluation of an effective partnership. *The Partnership Protocol* was designed for the physical activity and sport sector, although the guidelines and advice are transferable to other sectors. I hope this important work leads to more efficient board meetings, the development of responsible and effective partnerships, more resources for the sector, and healthy active lifestyles for all.

The Healthy Active Living and Obesity Research Group (HALO, www.haloresearch. ca) is located within the Children's Hospital of Eastern Ontario Research Institute (CHEO-RI, Ottawa, Canada), where it provides national leadership and research excellence in healthy active living for the prevention, management, and treatment of obesity in children and youth. Responding to the individual, familial, community, and societal call for help, the CHEO-RI made a strategic decision to create this center of excellence in healthy living and childhood obesity research. The HALO team is composed of a multidisciplinary group of research scientists, clinicians, research staff, administrative support, graduate and practicum students, postdoctoral fellows, medical interns, and residents. Working with local, provincial, and national partners and stakeholders, HALO has accepted the challenge to overcome the clinical and public health challenges of childhood obesity and inactivity and has a mission to preserve, enhance, and restore the health and wellness of our most precious resource, our children.

Active Healthy Kids Canada is a charitable organization that advocates the importance of physical activity for children and youth where they live, learn, and play (www. activehealthykids.ca). As a national leader in this area, Active Healthy Kids Canada advances knowledge to influence decision makers at all levels, from policy makers to parents, to increase the attention given to, investment in, and effective implementation of physical activity opportunities for all Canadian children and youth.

GLOBAL APPLICATION QUESTIONS

1. Strong evidence from around the globe indicates that not-for-profit organizations are facing increased competition and reduced government funding. In addition to partnerships, what strategies can these organizations implement to increase their revenues?

2. Dr. Tremblay speaks to the importance of *The Partnership Protocol*. How can researchers like Dr. Tremblay aid in convincing not-for-profits to use it?

3. Dr. Tremblay is well respected for his work characterizing the inactivity crisis in Canada. What other countries of the world are also facing an inactivity crisis?

Guidelines for Effective Partnerships

The Partnership Protocol offers a useful guide for public organizations to approach and assess effective partnership potential. Note as well that several other organizations have created guidelines for public and private organizational partnerships that may be useful within the scope of your organization, including two examples described here: (a) the Commonwealth Games Canada Partnership Filter and Application Toolkit and (b) the Research Centre for Sport in Canadian Society's Management Model for Sport and Physical Activity Partnerships.

Commonwealth Games Canada Partnership Filter and Application Toolkit

Van Kempen (2008) recommended that public partners use the Commonwealth Games Canada Partnership Filter and Application Toolkit to assess a private partner. Cousens et al. (2006) and van Kempen (2008) emphasized the importance of understanding the diverse goals, visions, and beliefs of each partner to be able to meet partnership expectations. The Partnership Filter and Application allows organizations to evaluate a potential partner based on questions relating to visions, values, readiness, driving forces, synergy, sustainability, links to local structures, long-term benefits, win–win benefits, and operating principles (Commonwealth Games Canada 2009). Partnerships can be strained or fail because of unclear roles and expectations, as well as inadequacies in employee training, time, communication, evaluation, and retention and termination strategies (Frisby, Thibault, and Kikulis 2004). Additionally, the Partnership Filter can assist in finding an appropriate partner. Weiermair, Peters, and Frehse (2008) stressed the importance of selecting the right partner—a partner who is willing to commit to long-term stability of the partnership's goals.

Research Centre for Sport in Canadian Society's Management Model for Sport and Physical Activity Partnerships

Researchers at the Centre for Sport in Canadian Society identified the challenge of developing partnerships, especially when the definition of partnership is so vague across sectors. Given the growth in partnership-based trend in sport aimed at increasing community physical activity levels especially in children, Parent and Harvey (2009) proposed a partnership framework to follow and evaluate a partnership from inception to its conclusion. Their proposal included three main aspects: antecedents, management, and evaluation of the partnership.

1. The antecedents included a determination of the project purposes, goals, and motives, taking into account the general environment (e.g., political, demographic, economic, sociocultural) and the task environment (e.g., customers, members, and fans; clubs; associations; agencies). The precursors should also include a review of partnership complementarity and fit while planning what type of partnership to pursue and how it will be governed.

2. The management of the partnership should be built on attributes of commitment, coordination, trust, organizational identity, organizational learning, mutuality, synergy, and staffing. Communication quality and

participation were deemed key to sharing information, and the decision-making structure needed to be clear and to have in place appropriate conflict resolution, power balance, and leadership strategies.

3. In the evaluation of the partnership, Parent and Harvey (2009) recommended that organizations examine the ongoing partnership process and immediate formative feedback that can improve the program in progress, the short-term effect of the partnership on participants, and the longer-term outcomes and satisfaction of participants and partners to evaluate the summative effectiveness and success of the partnership.

Conclusion

With the scarce resources allocated to sport, health, and physical activity organizations, partnering with businesses and corporations can fill the support gap, provide reciprocal, though perhaps not equal, benefits for both partners, and prevent further growth in the physical inactivity crisis. By sharing equity and being clear about your organization's goals, expectations, and expected risks, your partnership can draw on the right social and stakeholder support. A partnership built on honesty, trust, mutual respect, and transparency will be open to evaluation and reevaluation of the partnership as it grows and responds to the needs of each partner and the broader sport participants.

Building an effective partnership requires careful assessment of the best partnership fit in terms of shared goals and capacities, long-term commitments, champion leadership, and communication strategies, as well as how well each partner understands the potential risks and disconnect. Some challenges and conflict should be expected in building a relationship with a partner, but with clear and open communication, accountability, roles, and responsibilities, organizations can manage and move past the differences without tarnishing or slowing the partnership's momentum. Through regular monitoring and evaluation, the partnership can continue to grow and evolve and can potentially be renewed with increasing mutual partner benefits, which are increasingly reaped by people who improve their access or commitment to sport and physical activities that are central to the partnerships.

In part II, we will explore specific tactics to put the partnership guidelines into action in your organization. The emphasis will be on communicating effectively and building effective marketing messages in collaborative partnerships, sponsorship agreements, and philanthropy models.

Public–Private Partnership Strategies

Part I of the book was composed of two detailed chapters that provided the rationale and importance of public–private partnerships and shared guidelines about managing such partnerships in a responsible manner in the health, sport, and physical activity sectors. Chapter 1 laid the foundation for the book by outlining our view of partnerships and the way in which our experiences and empirical analyses led us to that understanding. Chapter 2 started by sharing *The Partnership Protocol,* a document that was based on extensive research and consultation (see appendix A for details on the research and consultation process).

We have taken the position that this book is in favor of partnerships but only if they are done in the right way (i.e., a responsible way). The caveat that partnerships must be done properly is fundamental to this book and to our view of partnerships. This leads us to part II of the book, which shares strategies and tactics related to finding, developing, implementing, and evaluating public–private partnerships in health, sport, and physical activity. Part II, Public–Private Partnership Strategies, includes chapters that address the key strategic areas in these partnerships, including marketing, sponsorship, fund-raising, philanthropy, role models and champions, and social responsibility. Each of these strategy areas has a chapter devoted to it in part II.

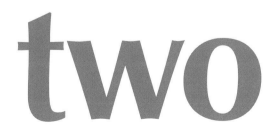

CHAPTER 3

Basics of Messaging and Marketing in Physical Activity and Health

Every time you walk through the grocery store, turn on your computer or TV, or open your newspaper, you are exposed to messages that are trying to reach your attention. These messages are designed and constructed by marketers. What are these marketers trying to achieve? How do these messages translate into your purchase decisions? How do the messages you see and hear affect your decisions to buy a product or make a change in your lifestyle?

An effective marketing strategy includes good internal communication. This attribute is key to bringing your organization's message to your targeted audiences and is critical to the way that people will accept, support, and participate in your program. In its simplest terms, communications theory applied to health, sport, and physical activity tells us that your messages first have to expose people to what it is that you are trying to convey, thereby helping generate awareness and knowledge about how your program fits in their life. But long before people can commit to changing their behavior in favor of a healthier one, they need to see and understand the significant value that the proposed change will have on their life. The role of marketing is to demonstrate to the targets the value to them of undertaking such a change. This value may be individual (a need or want) or societal (a change that will benefit the target as part of a better society).

Various tools, including web and social media, are available to marketers and managers to communicate their messages. Organizations can use these tools to interact with their partners and clients in an efficient way. The traditional "tools of inactivity" such as computers and TV that have often been a source of blame for our growing obesity crisis can in fact be effective modes of promoting physical activity, health, and sport to counteract this crisis. For example, social media is a way of delivering your messages to wider target groups that differ in age, gender, region, ethnicity, and culture. Studying your target audience and determining how you can most effectively deliver your message internally and externally to that audience is one of the keys to putting your communications strategy into action.

As presented in chapters 1 and 2, any interested organization, either private sector or public sector, should spend significant time at the onset of developing a partnership to find the right partner—an organization that has common goals and is willing to share resources and assets to form a strong partnership for a significant period. Partnerships that are short in duration, are one-dimensional in their benefits, and lack common goals are not successful for either partner.

A common marketing communications strategy between the partners to activate the partnership is a key component of any successful relationship between two organizations. Even in the best-intentioned partnerships, programs can (and often do) fail if they lack effective marketing plans to communicate with the populations that the partners hope to serve. In the case of physical activity, health, and sport partnership programs, these plans are often aimed at encouraging behavioral change (e.g., join our club, cut down your salt, bike to work, practice safe sex), but the organizations involved in the partnership cannot achieve the sought changes unless they have a strong, collaborative communications strategy to build awareness in their target audiences and, later, to encourage some of those people (the targets) to get on board with the program.

Social media tools can help organizations involved in a partnership deliver their messages, as well as act as a source of secondary research to help them obtain valuable information as people contribute to online blogs or web discussion boards about the direction and effect of the partnership and its related programs. These benefits of online elements are relatively new in health promotion, because TV and computers were traditionally seen as tools of inactivity that took time away from healthy and active pursuits. But many health professionals, educators, researchers, and organizations are now starting to see ways to use new technology to promote physical activity and fitness across wide audience spectrums. Indeed, the two principal benefits of efficient reach and secondary research are profound in this regard. For small organizations, like many not-for-profits in health, sport, and physical activity, the ability to reach members, build awareness in other markets, and achieve media coverage is now possible (although still challenging) where it once was financially impossible. With respect to market research, an entire methodology, known as netnography (Kozinets 2002), has developed that allows researchers to use online data from blogs, chats, and other social media platforms as a source of data to learn more about markets, products, and opportunities.

Importance of a Good Communications Strategy

Many partnerships seek to increase physical activity, healthy behaviors, and sport participation. Thus, these outcomes are often the goal of the partnership and the accompanying messages. These types of partnerships are the focus of this book. When sport is an element of the partnership, it can also act as a tool to communicate another often more important message (e.g., consider Right To Play's use of sport to promote peace building, integration, and self-confidence in youth). Pegoraro et al. (2010) emphasize this point, noting that sport is "a corporate marketing tool [that] provides increased flexibility, broad reach, and high levels of brand and corporate exposure" (p. 1454). This idea also applies to partnerships based on health and physical activity, in which health (e.g., the Canadian Mental Health Association's implementation of a program to reduce the negative stigma around mental health) or physical activity (e.g., ParticipACTION's SOGO active program) can act as tools to support communications efforts. Whether physical activity, health, or sport is the goal of the message, or whether it is the medium of the message (e.g., advertising through sport, sport-based sponsorship), both private-sector and public-sector partners must be effective story tellers for their messages to reach their target audiences.

One of the stages of *The Partnership Protocol* that was presented in chapter 2 includes a commitment to establishing a communications strategy and building a relationship framework to engage stakeholders and tell a story. The research process undertaken (see appendix A) to develop *The Partnership Protocol* included numerous expert consultations with a consensus expressed around the vital importance of communicating the benefits of any public–private partnership both internally and externally. Consider even groundbreaking results from rigorous research; despite the importance of the conclusions, the research is not important or appreciated until it is communicated and translated to health professionals, educators, and finally individuals and their families. The analogy holds well for partnerships. To grow knowledge of their use and importance, positive experience must be widely communicated. Thus, the message, its reach, and the way that people interpret and use your partnership's message are crucial to the success of your partnership.

Communications Strategies

Within a partnership, two main communications strategies should be considered. The first is a plan to share information about the partnership internally, within your own organization and with your partners. With a good internal communications strategy in place, you can then reach out externally to begin to build and share your message in hopes of successfully implementing your partnership's goals and objectives. Partners should collaborate in planning their communications strategies at the onset of the partnership, considering each other's policies, procedures, needs, and objectives (UN 2007). In summary, the organizations involved in any partnership need to plan both an internal and an external communications plan.

Successful partnerships are built on mutual understanding and clear goals and objectives. A strong internal communications plan that considers how best to share and distribute information among, within, and between partners is a necessary part of good partnership management. Open and clear messages drum up internal support for the partnership, help to identify opportunities or gaps, and can create a sense of employee pride and engagement that can be expressed through employee participation or volunteering in a partnership fitness or health program. Between partners, good communication can eliminate some of the misunderstandings that lead to program failure. Internal communication relies on having clear leadership in each organization, including identified people who maintain regular contact (by phone, e-mail, social media tools, or in person) as the partnership progresses. These leaders and their teams should understand how to manage and promote the partnership internally, which can inspire increased internal support for the partnership and be a good basis on which to take the message external.

A good external communications strategy is crucial to the partnership's success. It will determine how much the public is willing to buy into the partnership. External communications should address how the partnership goals can benefit the public (e.g., contributing to increased health) and aim to increase the demand in the programs (Vail 2007). In essence, a partnership is never completed until the details are shared with citizens and private businesses or organizations that will use the programs; they need to be sold on the process and outcome of the partnership (e.g., the program, the facility, or the product created) (Rosentraub and Swindell 2009). In Vail's (2007) examination of Tennis Canada's partnerships, communication action aimed to introduce more people to tennis in local communities through rallies and meetings with private community and tennis leaders. Like internal communications plans, external communication messages can increase support for the partnership, which can motivate more people to contribute volunteer hours or donations.

In creating a communications plan, partners must consider accountability and transparency to protect public interests. Recently, as Hodge and Greve (2007) explained, public–private partnerships have been criticized for low communication and transparency, which can decrease public confidence in the partnerships. To increase communication and transparency in a public–private soccer stadium project in Slovenia, the public partner maintained a public online system to explain details of the partnership and allowed the submission of anonymous questions (Ferk and Ferk 2008). Answers were provided in a timely manner by e-mail to interested parties. Each partner should be ready to answer to conflicting pressure from the media. Communications and press release strategies should be clarified at the beginning of the partnership, and all partner-to-partner negotiations should be kept confidential until the communications strategy is in place (Rosentraub and Swindell 2009).

Governments, Alliances, and Partnerships

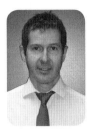

Craig Larsen
Executive Director, Chronic Disease Prevention Alliance of Canada

BIO

Craig has worked in the health sector for 23 years in policy, research, and practice domains. After working for several years in acute and palliative nursing, he moved into administration and participated in the implementation of health care regionalization in British Columbia. Working as a policy consultant at the Health Association of BC, Craig facilitated a number of collaborative projects that brought together representatives from a wide range of sectors and stakeholder groups. These projects included feedback to government on policies and programs and implementation of accountability systems for health authorities. Craig managed the inaugural iteration of the Canadian Institutes of Health Research's Institute of Health Services and Policy Research and helped develop and support research-funding programs. Currently, Craig is executive director at the Chronic Disease Prevention Alliance of Canada, which focuses on childhood obesity and food security.

CHRONIC DISEASE PREVENTION ALLIANCE OF CANADA (CDPAC)

CDPAC is an alliance of 10 national NGOs (Canadian Alliance on Mental Illness and Mental Health, Canadian Cancer Society, Canadian Council for Tobacco Control, Canadian Diabetes Association, Canadian Public Health Association, Coalition for Active Living, Dietitians of Canada, Heart and Stroke Foundation of Canada, the Kidney Foundation of Canada, and YMCA Canada) who agree that some aspects of their respective mandates can be done more effectively by working together in alliance.

One senior-level representative from each member organization is appointed by his or her organization to sit on the CDPAC Alliance, which functions similarly to a board of directors. The alliance sets the overall strategic direction for the organization (e.g., topic areas, priorities). Each member organization contributes resources as well, both financial and in-kind in the form of project work and operational support services.

Another major arm of our partnership is the Network of Provincial and Territorial Alliances, created by CDPAC to provide a forum for key players in healthy living at the provincial and territorial levels to link, share, and collaborate. Two representatives from these local alliances sit at the CDPAC Alliance table and participate in CDPAC business on behalf of the overall network.

Although CDPAC has just two employees, including me, we are in fact a partnership involving many people. Numerous employees from member organizations participate in our collective work, as do many people from the network. We don't currently have private-sector participation in the CDPAC partnership, but we do liaise with various industry representatives on a project basis as appropriate.

CDPAC's mandate comprises three main streams:

1. Advocacy—influencing public policy related to chronic disease prevention in priority topic areas
2. Knowledge development and exchange—supporting the creation and dissemination of evidence and information to provide a rational basis for our advocacy portfolios
3. Facilitating an integrated approach to chronic disease prevention—functioning as both a forum and a catalyst for alliance members and players in other organizations and sectors to work together for chronic disease prevention

My role as executive director is to provide facilitative and operational leadership for fulfillment of this mandate.

It is under the second point, knowledge development and exchange, and the third, integrated approach, that the idea of partnership becomes particularly meaningful to CDPAC. We've chosen to work in partnership because several of the key risk factors associated with member organizations' respective mandates are common across the broad alliance (such as nutritional practices and physical activity levels). As mentioned earlier, we know that we can do a better job of influencing the policy environment by working together.

Given the strong links between obesity (which is largely a consequence of food and beverage consumption patterns and activity levels) and several cancers and chronic diseases, we think that it is important to set our sights upstream. Childhood obesity is therefore a priority area for action by CDPAC.

MARKETING IN HEALTH

CDPAC is trying to change the Canadian landscape around the marketing of unhealthy foods and beverages to children. Our advocacy work is primarily at the federal government level. The alliance worked together to develop a policy position, and delegations from the alliance now meet with ministers and senior government officials to review the evidence linking marketing and childhood obesity and to deliver our policy recommendations—making a plea for control and regulation of marketing to kids across Canada. The province of Quebec is one of the few places in the world that has taken a regulatory approach, and we're seeing that it can work.

In addition to our federal-level lobbying, we also convene pan-Canadian conferences, webinars, and education campaigns directed at a broader range of stakeholders such as public health workers, government personnel, and the academic sector to advance awareness and evidence of the links between factors such as marketing and

(continued) ▶

(continued) ▶

sugar-sweetened beverage consumption and obesity. The overall aim of our efforts in this regard is to increase awareness and capacity to take action on childhood obesity. In turn, this contributes to a groundswell of public support for our advocacy.

At present, CDPAC does not directly target consumers (families and parents) in its campaigns and activities. But we have recently partnered with three other organizations to explore the potential for building in Canada something like the so-called Parent's Jury program in Australia. It is directed at, and essentially run by, parents. One of its interesting tactics is to hold annual "fame and shame" awards in which parents nominate and vote for food and beverage organizations that are doing progressive marketing to support better health (fame) and those that are being particularly damaging in terms of influencing unhealthy food and beverage choices by kids (shame).

IMPORTANCE OF PARTNERSHIPS

In my view, wider-reaching partnerships are vital to continued growth and progress in Canada's chronic disease prevention domain. Partnerships between NGO organizations such as CDPAC and other sectors outside the health care and chronic disease prevention arenas will play an increasingly important role. I mentioned, for example, that insufficient activity levels are a major contributor to obesity. We have to look at the various reasons why people are not more active and address those reasons. We know that the web of causation is complex and multifaceted. Therefore, we have to be prepared to take action at many levels and across many sectors. New forms of partnership are needed so that greater connectivity can be achieved between those who understand the consequences of factors such as a poorly designed community and the urban planners and municipalities who are responsible for such decisions.

Reflecting on my 26 years in various roles within the policy realm, I have identified numerous critical success factors for effective partnerships. Of the lessons that I have learned, I believe the most important is the need for trusted relationships. Trust develops through communication. All partners must develop and maintain a shared understanding of objectives, roles, and responsibilities. Attaining this objective depends on regular communication that is clear and purposeful. You need to stay in touch. As everyone knows, nothing beats in-person, face-to-face connections at least once or twice per year. But in between, you have to maintain the trusted relationship by carefully protecting sufficient calendar time for regular connectivity through electronic or other means. For me, that is a critical piece.

GLOBAL APPLICATION QUESTIONS

1. Larsen discusses alliances amongst governments. How important do you think these are and why?

2. Should these alliances be allowed to partner with for-profit corporations? If so, are there any restrictions that you would suggest? If not, why not?

3. Larsen notes that CDPAC does not directly target consumers in its campaigns and activities, but how does CDPAC engage families and parents in their work?

Marketing for Behavioral Change

The goal of many partnerships in physical activity, sport, and health is to influence and change the decisions and behaviors of individuals. Partnerships may aim to increase participation in a grassroots sport, persuade people to make better food choices, or motivate them to commit to a walking program. To influence the individual, the partnership needs to be able to translate the marketing message from strategy into behavioral change. Craig et al. (2007) examined the messaging variables aimed to increase walking in adults as part of the Canada on the Move (COTM) initiative. A partnership between the Canadian Institutes of Health Research and Kellogg Canada, the 2004 program distributed pedometers in cereal boxes and promoted walking for health through a mass media campaign and the accompanying slogan "Donate your steps to health research" (Craig et al. 2007). The back of Kellogg's Special K cereals explained the use of the pedometer in helping people achieve and maintain healthy body weight. The campaign messaging targeted six variables, concluding with behavioral change. First, the COTM aimed to *expose* people (breakfast cereal consumers) to the importance of health. The second goal was to generate *awareness* of the benefits of the "Add 2,000 steps" message. Third, the campaign wanted to create better *knowledge* about walking and using pedometers, and fourth, it sought to draw *attention* to the importance of walking in a person's life. Fifth, by increasing awareness, knowledge, and attention, the campaign hoped to influence people's *intentions*. Finally, the campaign encouraged the translation of those intentions into *behavioral change* (specifically, adding 2,000 steps per day) (see table 3.1). In one year, the COTM program was successful at increasing walking by 13 percent in adults who owned a pedometer and who were aware of the partnership's message. The tagline "Donate your steps to health research" was an appealing message that fit with Canadian adults' concern for overall health and desire to be altruistic, and the pedometer and online monitoring system was an "opportunity for participating in immediate and reinforcing behaviour" (Craig et al. 2007, p. 411).

TABLE 3.1   Six Variables for Messages to Inspire Behavioral Change

Variable	Intended result
Exposure	Expose a target participant or group to the partnership's message or story
Awareness	Generate a sense of awareness about the partnership's personal or societal value
Knowledge	Transfer knowledge about the partnership goals and objectives
Attention	Bring into attention how the partnership could benefit the participant or target group
Intention	Create intention for change
Behavior change	Complete transformative change to a more healthy behavior

Based on Craig, Tudor-Locke, and Mauman 2007.

A Private Sector View on Partnerships

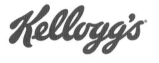

Reprinted, by permission, from Kellogg Company.

Christine Lowry
Vice President, International Nutrition, Kellogg Company
Vice President, Nutrition and Corporate Affairs, Kellogg Canada Inc.

BIO

Christine Lowry was appointed vice president of international nutrition, Kellogg Company, and vice president of nutrition and corporate affairs, Kellogg Canada Inc. in June 2011. Before being appointed to these positions, she served as Kellogg Canada's vice president of nutrition, government, and corporate affairs.

Ms. Lowry joined the company as a nutritionist in 1983 and since then has held several leadership positions with the company, including manager of strategic planning, chair of Kellogg Company's global nutrition team, and vice president of global nutrition marketing.

In her current role as vice president, international nutrition, Kellogg Company, Ms. Lowry provides global coordination of the nutrition marketing function and represents Kellogg with international nutrition organizations such as the World Health Organization. As vice president, nutrition and corporate affairs, Kellogg Canada, she is responsible for nutrition science and regulatory affairs, nutrition marketing, consumer and quality services, corporate communications, and government and public affairs for the Canadian business.

An active member of Food & Consumer Products of Canada (FCPC) on issues relating to food and nutrition policy, she was also a member of the Grocery Manufacturers of America's Food, Health and Strategy Group.

She has served on the advisory boards for Corus Television's YTV and Treehouse TV and is past chair of Concerned Children's Advertisers and a former executive member of the board. She is also the past vice-chairman of the Canadian Council of Food and Nutrition, is a former member of the board of directors of Dietitians of Canada, and has served on the executive committee of the National Institute of Nutrition.

Ms. Lowry received a bachelor's degree in human nutrition from the University of Guelph in Guelph, Ontario, and a master's degree in community nutrition from the University of Manitoba in Winnipeg, Manitoba. Ms. Lowry is a registered dietitian and a member of the Ontario College of Dietitians and the Dietitians of Canada.

Ms. Lowry was born in Niagara Falls, Ontario. She and her husband, Douglas, reside in Burlington, Ontario. They have two children.

MY VIEW ON PARTNERSHIPS

I've been at Kellogg for 28 years and have been involved in many different partnership projects over the years. In an early partnership, we worked with the Canadian

Cancer Society to deliver messages about the impact of low-fat dietary consumption in lowering cancer risks. In later years, we partnered with Health Canada and the Nova Scotia Heart Health Programme to promote the health benefits of breakfast. We also partnered with the Canadian Institutes of Health Research (CIHR) to promote free pedometers in boxes of Special K cereal and encourage Canadians to start walking and registering their commitments. Kellogg seeks out partners and, in some cases, is approached by numerous organizations that view us as a natural partner in supporting health initiatives. For example, Health Canada was delighted when we started printing the Canada Food Guide on cereal boxes because it had the potential to reach every Canadian household, a much more significant reach than could have been achieved by Health Canada without our partnership. Moreover, Kellogg products are seen as welcoming and comforting, and consumers have confidence in our health messages.

PARTNERSHIPS TO BENEFIT OUR CONSUMERS

As an industry member of FCPC, we've been working in partnership with Health Canada to create generic health messages on the back of food items to educate consumers about how to read nutritional labels. This is an example in which the majority of the food industry (over 34 food manufacturers and food services) has engaged in a partnership with Health Canada to meet the needs of consumers and help them interpret information to make food choices relevant to their personal nutritional needs. Launched in October 2010, the partnership has been able to create generic and user-friendly messages about what daily values (DV) percentage means across the board in the food industry and how to interpret the information.

A KELLOGG CANADA PARTNERSHIP IN ACTION

Over the course of our 11-year partnership with the Dietitians of Canada, we have worked to bring well-respected expert speakers to deliver educational programming for health professionals at the annual Kellogg Nutrition Symposium (KNS). This event is held annually within the national Dietitians of Canada Conference, which is rotated among cities across Canada. The symposium brings together health and nutritional professionals, government, educators, and industry representatives to provide relevant information on health and nutrition issues based on current educational needs and trends. We colead and sponsor the symposium's breakfast, and Kellogg is the only food company to have this type of formal relationship with the Dietitians of Canada. Our partnership allows them to offer a caliber of speakers that they could not otherwise afford, thereby helping them attract a greater audience to their national conference. We seek speakers who can share research and recommendations related to topics such as the benefits of breakfast cereal consumption by children, updates to the U.S. dietary guidelines, the latest science exploring the effects of vitamin D, and the importance of increasing fiber intake. We try to help health professionals stay current and build our program based on scientific progress and feedback from previous symposiums.

(continued) ▶

(continued) ▶

OUR CONSISTENT MESSAGE: PROMOTING HEALTH AND WELLNESS

Kellogg is consistent in its message to health professionals and consumers regarding the facts behind the health contribution of breakfast cereals in supporting healthy lifestyles and a healthy body mass index. We are also consistent in our message to these stakeholder groups about our focus on the overall health and wellness of the population. In keeping with our company's more than 100-year heritage of nutrition leadership, our most important corporate giving priorities are focused on the two areas where we believe we can make the biggest impact. First, we work to address hunger through our partnerships with food banks and breakfast clubs. Second, we support programs that seek to reduce the risk of obesity by promoting healthy eating and physical activity. Our efforts in Canada are mirrored in other Kellogg core markets including Australia, France, Mexico, the United Kingdom, and the United States.

ADVICE FOR BUILDING SUCCESSFUL PARTNERSHIPS

Imagine two intersecting circles, each representing a prospective partner. The intersecting sweet spot is the beginning of a partnership, where our values and objectives converge. We can build from there. We need to ask ourselves how that sweet spot translates into developing a partnership and a user-friendly, executable contract. Unlike a marriage, the partnership needs a clear definition of how it ends before it begins. At the onset the partnership seems ideal, but it's important to think about how difference of opinions, expectations, and values would be dealt with before the partnership progresses forward. Who breaks the tie? Thinking through the partnership from beginning to end is a crucial piece that should not be overlooked in the excitement of a blossoming relationship.

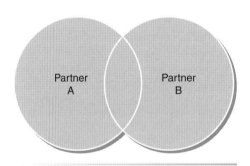

Building from the sweet spot.

GLOBAL APPLICATION QUESTIONS

1. Lowry discusses a number of public-sector partners that she has partnered with over the years. Describe, in your view, why Kellogg would partner with these organizations.

2. In her perspective, Lowry stresses the importance of consistent messaging. Why is this important for a private-sector partner?

3. Describe what Lowry means by the sweet spot.

Communicating Through Social Media

Social media is a tool that partners can use for both internal and external communication purposes. Social media is made up of constantly growing user-generated interactive conversations to build relationships, stakeholders, and support through online websites. Marketing through social media reflects a willingness to listen to consumer needs and wants to develop and modify programs accordingly (Bryant et al. 2001). Indeed, it allows for rapid feedback and alterations to programs based on that feedback. Marketing approaches based on social media have been used in physical activity and sport programming to increase target group enrollment, enhance program delivery, raise satisfaction levels of participants and staff, increase fan support and enhance fan experience, and boost overall community outreach (see Bryant et al. 2001; Dharod et al. 2011; Grier and Bryant 2005; Waters et al. 2011). Web-based meetings can also be used as a way to find and develop partnerships (see Kruger et al. 2011). Many not-for-profit and business organizations use social media websites to increase collaboration with consumers and receive authentic and dynamic feedback, such as www.sogoactive.com, where ParticipACTION hosts young people who can access information, participate in group chats, keep tabs on their activity levels, design activity programs, and read motivating testimonials. O'Reilly and Foster (2010) detailed other avenues such as, (a) life-streaming or social networking websites that produce user-generated profiles and contributions (e.g., Facebook, Twitter, YouTube); (b) social news-sharing sites that offer user rankings based on unique or usefulness appeal (e.g., Digg, Delicious, Reddit); (c) personal or business blogs and podcasts to provide readers regular access to information and commentary. Sport participation programs are now common in cities around the globe. The specific activities of these programs include Bike to Work Weeks, Walk to Work Days, Car Pools, and Get Up Get Active Campaigns. In these examples, cities are using community awareness strategies to draw increased message awareness, support, and participation. A typical four-step strategic process towards online success involves (1) research to understand how your community accesses information and uses social media, (2) articulation of your online goals, (3) articulation of a community engagement strategy (e.g., blog, contest, website, social media platform), and (4) development of a long-term plan to implement.

Social media can bring multiple minds to a project and inform the partnership of user needs and wants. Organizations should also realize that, as Waters et al. (2011) reminded us, social media "messages

> There is perhaps no group that stands to benefit more from the pervasiveness of social media than nonprofits.
>
> Simon Mainwaring (2011)

are constantly changing and being shaped by those outside the organization" (p. 167). With increased external public feedback that is out of the partners' control, including feedback from competitors, organizations need to plan how they will deal with dissenting opinions and negative comments while still respecting the openness desired in social media participation. In addition, measuring the full impact of social media and networking is difficult, especially in terms of measuring the return on investment (Waters et al. 2011). Despite the challenges, most organizations (public and private) see social media as part of the new norm in creating relationships with consumers and program participants.

According to Mainwaring (2011), the proliferation of social media has given not-for-profit organizations a useful and easy way to generate greater awareness about their goals and objectives. Because private businesses want to engage in more meaningful ways with their clients, they often look to a partnership with a not-for-profit to express their core values. Capitalism is changing because more consumers want to see a company's profit tied to social change and a good cause. The public not-for-profit group must therefore be able to "market" their single-message brand and demonstrate the distinct benefits that businesses can obtain through the partnership. Social media facilitates communication to the consumer, but amidst competing social interests, not-for-profit organizations need to be more creative in their communications strategies to draw interest, funding, and long-term results (Mainwaring 2011). *Runner's World* magazine, in partnership with Crowdrise (a unique online fund-raising platform that incorporates crowd sourcing and social networking through champions like actor Edward Norton), has created the Outrunning Cancer program. Through *Runner's World* e-mails and websites, runners are encouraged to make their race or training count by choosing a cancer charity to support; the platform makes it easy for runners to donate to an organization of their choice or to start their own fund-raiser.

Social-media-based marketing can be a tool to deliver messages about a partnership to broader audiences, but the rise in social media and crowd sourcing also allows people (i.e., the target audiences) to become an integral part of building a partnership. Indeed, input from prospective clients can help partners identify pressing needs and set the partnership objectives. Prospective clients can also become agents who are able to extend the reach of the partnership so that programs can be shaped and melded through the collaboration and contributions of people worldwide. For example, in developing the Fiat Miao car in Brazil, the marketing firm AgênciaClick Isobar and Fiat Brazil collected input from Internet crowd sourcing, compiling contributions from over 17,000 people in 160 countries (Houpt 2011). The crowd-sourcing efforts are a reflection of the way that people are being thought of as a new and important partner, a partner that can help build and generate excitement about the partnership.

Harnessing Tools of Inactivity to Promote Physical Activity

Using social media to communicate the goals of the partnership to the target audience is inherently challenging because the message relies on attracting participants through modes that are already increasing levels of sedentary leisure-time activities in young people, such as television viewing, video games, and personal computing (Berger et al. 2008). According to People Meter, in 2008–2009 males between 12 and 17 were spending an average of 24.3 hours in front of a screen per week and females between 12 and 17 were spending 23.6 hours. Given this context, organizations have the challenge of engaging the target audience, especially young people, in physical activity, healthy behaviors, and sport participation through social media without contributing to the increasing screen time that is linked to poor health. Increased screen activities and "computer addiction" compete for the scarce time needed to participate in physical activities and sport, particularly among adolescents (Berger et al. 2008).

Recently, a trend has developed to use screen activities and portable technology to encourage rather than compete with physical activities. For example, programs like Cardio Cinema allow participants to watch television or movies while working out on a treadmill (Berger et al. 2008). Similarly, iPod–Nike strength and endurance tracks mix music with a voiceover that encourage a set amount of warm-up, varied intensity, and recovery cool-down for runners. An added benefit is that runners are able to take the workout anywhere and use GPS monitors to track run time, distance, and intensity by a computer program. If screen time and multitasking is part of adolescent culture, then effective delivery of partnership programs can use these tools to promote physical activity among young people.

The Learn to Camp at Ontario Parks program, a partnership between Ontario Parks, the Ontario Ministry of Natural Resources, and private companies Coleman, Foodland, and Pepsi, offers an online option to help visitors prepare for an active outdoor adventure (Ontario Parks 2011). The program guides users through four stages: (1) Planning Ahead includes a preparation checklist and advice about meals and gear; (2) Setting Up Your Campsite directs prospective campers through the registration and arrival process to the practical side of setting up a tent and camp kitchen; (3) Tips for Life at Camp provides details about safe, fun, clean, and "green" camping with dogs and children; (4) Packing Up Your Campsite introduces the concept of leave-no-trace camping and packing up and storing gear to get ready for the next adventure. The program takes advantage of the availability and interest in screen time to promote future active participation in camping activities with direct links to book online camping reservations. The Learn to Camp at

Ontario Parks partnership markets camping through a useful and informative website for users, and it is teamed with in-person overnight camping options with full equipment and free community sessions.

Communicating Across Cultures

With rising immigration rates and growing diversity in cities and countries around the globe, communication messages must increasingly focus on how programs and marketing messages will appeal to diverse cultural groups, in terms of both language and culturally relevant content. The growing ethnic diversity in cities worldwide has not been accompanied by an increase in culturally appropriate physical activity programming for low-income, minority, and underserved populations (Cheadle et al. 2010). Similar arguments can be made for other healthy behaviors and sport participation (Berger et al., 2008). According to Beaulac et al. (2010), community members "who are socially or economically disadvantaged participate significantly less in physical activity" especially in youth (p. 62). Attracting underrepresented groups to physical activity, health, and sport programs requires a communications strategy that reaches beyond traditional venues (e.g., recreation centers) to other community organizations including ethnic community associations, faith groups, and local business associations (Cheadle et al. 2010). For example, Beaulac et al. (2010) described the example of a community-based hip-hop dance program that targeted disadvantaged youth and successfully crossed ethnocultural lines in a disadvantaged area in South-East Ottawa, Canada. The program was free, noncompetitive, and supervised in an easily accessible location, and it offered incentives for participation. In the short term, the program aimed to increase physical, psychological, and social wellness; self-identity; and social relationships. Longer term objectives were to reduce violent behaviors, improve academic attendance and results, and foster positive community engagement (Beaulac et al. 2010). The program received positive community and parent feedback and was built on appropriate consultation with the targeted cultural and youth groups. The key learning from this case is that linking with nontraditional groups and nurturing coalitions amongst partners that reach across cultural and age barriers can increase program participation and support. A reasonable expectation is that approaches like this can work in many areas of health, sport, and physical activity to reach the ever-diversifying populations of developed countries.

Given the ever-changing and highly specialized reality of social media, we asked an expert—Chuck Hamilton, social learning leader at IBM's Center for Advanced Learning—to summarize for us (see Executive Perspective).

Key Elements of Messaging and Marketing in Physical Activity and Health

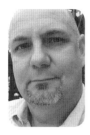

Chuck Hamilton
Social Learning Leader, IBM Center for Advanced Learning

BIO

Chuck Hamilton is a social media solutions leader in IBM's Center for Advanced Learning. Before taking this post, Chuck was the learning and new media solution lead for IBM's 3D Internet EBO and leader of a program called IBM@Play. Chuck is also an associate instructor for the Master of Digital Media Program at the Centre for Digital Media in Vancouver, Canada. Articles about Chuck's work have appeared in *Fast Company*, *Talent Management* magazine, *Meetings and Incentive* magazine, the *Wall Street Journal*, *Canadian Business*, and the *Globe and Mail*.

WHEN CHANGE COMES QUIETLY—HOW SOCIAL MEDIA AND CONNECTED HUMAN CAPITAL ARE CHANGING JUST ABOUT EVERYTHING

When sweeping and impactful changes occur—the sort of changes or trends that affect many lives, workplaces, or even mankind as a whole—we almost always see the professed change surrounded by superlatives intended to emphasize its importance. Words like *transformational*, *disruptive*, *unparalleled*, and *game changing* are common examples, signaling that an important shift is underway (or has already happened), and we had better pay close attention. Global warming and the global economic crisis are recent examples of sweeping changes that have captured our attention and spawned a number of independent and group actions.

Some sweeping changes, however, come quietly, too quickly, or just slip in under our radar, either eluding us or missing our mind space altogether. For these stealthy trends, superlatives and hype seem absent, and we are unable predict the looming opportunity. Eventually these seemingly subtly formed messages hit us in waves, coming from long off shore to hit us in the knees and knock us back a few paces, thereby demanding our attention. This is the sort of change that saw the number of mobile phone subscriptions reach 4.6 billion worldwide by 2010, a number that was expected to increase to 5 billion by the start of 2011. In fact, although mobile phone penetration grew 76.2 percent in 2010, fixed telephone lines dropped to 17.3 percent penetration worldwide. Although the arrival of the mobile wave seemed predictable and many of us are among the billions of subscribers, most of us did not imagine

(continued) ▶

(continued) ▶

that our home phone (landline) and Internet access would become nearly obsolete overnight. Did we really see the surge coming in so quickly? Did we really understand that this technology would change the way that we work, live, play, walk, and talk? Tweet me if you think that you were ready!

THE WAY THAT WE CONNECT AND ENGAGE

Another largely unobserved yet equally disruptive change is occurring in the way that humans connect, engage, and participate today. Most of us have not seen this wave coming, nor do we understand the opportunities flowing from the phenomenon. This shift is led and supported by the adoption of social media technology, mixed with a new collaborative attitude that has already resulted in a whole new era of human connectedness—a global stage for more change. Many people are missing this wave, and those who don't get it will quickly fall into another digital divide far more complex than the lack of affordable or scalable technology that we sensed 15 years ago.

If you think that by social media we mean Facebook (more than 750 million active users), Twitter (175 million accounts), LinkedIn (over 100 million users), Foursquare (725,000 users, 22 million check-ins), and Qzone (China's largest social network with 637 million active accounts), you would be right, but you would be wrong to believe that the human connectedness story ends there. In fact, these tools and literally thousands more (see the Conversation Prism V2.0 by Brian Solis) merely initiate the global conversation.

"As you read this and at every moment, in every day people are gathering, collaborating and connecting to work, learn and create new products and services without leadership direction to do so" (Bingham and Conner, 2010). We (the connected we) are learning to play together on a massive scale, finding deeper and more valuable social interactions every day. We are leveraging a host of social media tools and collaborative tactics, undaunted by geography, hierarchy, or business function. Our path is supported by people interacting with many other people imbued with a new spirit of participation, conversation, community, connectedness, and transparency. This new value is already more evenly distributed than at any other point in our evolution—afforded to every person logged in and open to invitation.

Whether you have hot new idea for a T-shirt and need someone to create it, rate it, and sell it for you (Threadless) or are leveraging crowds of experts and amateurs in globally disparate communities for innovation in new products and services (InnoCentive), you can make it happen with a little help from your online-connected friends. Whether your goal is to gain better understanding of a subject like trapeze and aerial skills or a specific chemotherapy treatment that others are using in brain tumor cases (PatientsLikeMe), you can find these communities of support and work your own magic.

On July 6, 2011, U.S. president Barack Obama hosted a live Twitter @The White House Town Hall event in which over 70,000 tweets were sent to the president either through the #AskObama hashtag or by mentioning the @townhall username. Topics included job creation, the economy, housing, and even the legalization of marijuana, all online, over a day of national collaboration and exchange with the Twitter universe. Were you there? Whether you are 10 or 110 years old, you can participate in similar town halls with no intervening hierarchy to obstruct your contribution. If you can log in and be identified, you are in the discussion. This pattern of inclusion is changing the fabric of public consultation, civic responsibility, and coordinated human action the world over.

To be a valued contributor in this storm of global connectedness, you need to understand how to use well-tested and distinguishing virtual characteristics to your advantage. Three of the most dynamic facets known by virtual collaborators are (a) trust—being a trusted, rated, ranked, and always respected source; (b) authenticity—being the genuine article, the "real you," an unencumbered and open virtual self; and (c) presence—being committed to be there, participating, producing, and consuming in the context of everyone else in the communities that you frequent. Savvy social players wield these characteristics like swords, cutting through the clutter and ambiguity of many virtual communities.

The changes described here are big, the sort of disruptive changes that we discussed earlier, ripe with unparalleled opportunity and freedom. An extraordinary opportunity has been firmly placed in the hands of those individuals, groups, and communities that care to leverage the connectedness to their advantage.

WHAT CHANGED?

If you look closely at the overarching social trends affecting human connection today compared with even five years ago, four prevalent themes emerge. Individually these themes are easily recognized (and might not seem influential), but combined they point toward a socially connected culture. Participants in this new culture learn that connectedness, combined with action, can represent a rich opportunity to share wisdom globally. The four connected themes are the following:

1. Ever-wider Internet adoption supported by far less expensive connection tools. Access to the Internet and the wealth of its resources has grown substantially in the past five years. The number of Internet users rose to 2.4 billion in 2012, or about 24% of the world's population (Internet World Stats 2012). This growth in demand combined with literally thousands of new, often free services (like Skype, Twitter, Foursquare, Facebook, and so on) buoys the producer–consumer community, demonstrating that true virtual work is not only a possibility but a part of everyday life.

2. Shared, inexpensive, and well-coordinated production. The emergence of tools, techniques, and inexpensive modes of production for the creation of many different things creates a powerful opportunity. This production can be either wholly virtual (creation of an entire online meeting space) or part of the process for creating something for real-world consumption (such as the Toyota Scion mod culture or the Pepsi Refresh Challenge).

(continued) ▶

(continued) ►

3. The emergence of a highly visible and level playing field. A virtual or physical place has developed where, across geography and culture, amateurs and professionals can commingle, cocreate, produce, and consume. At the same time, people can also leverage their crowd strength to teach, lead, and interact in a new many-to-many model.

4. The evolution and efficient organization of community voice. Perhaps the biggest and most significant shift is the creation of a community of communities that has a strong voice in everything from purchasing decisions and world governance to health care tips. Well-organized and moderated communities wield power and influence, ensuring that the crowd voice is now enabled as part of any important strategy. We are learning that although like-minded connectedness is highly desirable, diversity can also bring huge new opportunities and innovation to communities everywhere. This notion of a greater value through togetherness is old news in a way, as if we have gone back to an earlier era with an everyone-is-welcome-here attitude.

Author Clay Shirky (2010) offers one of the best summaries of opportunity represented by these major shifts in his compelling book *Cognitive Surplus—Creativity and Generosity in a Connected Age*. Shirky suggests,

> More value can be gotten out of voluntary participation than anyone previously imagined, thanks to improvements in our ability to connect with one another and improvements in our imagination of what is possible from such participation. We are emerging from an era of theory-induced blindness in which we thought sharing (and most nonmarket interaction) was inherently limited to small, tight-knit groups.

COORDINATED VOICES CAN MAKE SOMETHING HAPPEN!

This quiet, yet colossal, change in the way that humans connect with one another is in an early stage. But the waves have already hit many shores, and we all need to join the flow. Go out and make a new virtual friend today, join an online community, and begin to collect and coordinate a voice that can make something happen. Together we have the opportunity to make our planet just a little smarter. Trust us. There are plenty of friends waiting to connect with you.

GLOBAL APPLICATION QUESTIONS

1. Why is social media important for a public-sector partner?
2. Why is social media important for a private-sector partner?
3. Hamilton brings forth the notion of global connectedness. Describe what he means.

Conclusion

A partnership is only as good as its communications strategy, both internal and external. Without good messages between partners and to your clients or audiences, your program may not reach the people that you hope to influence. As with any marketing program, inefficient use of resources to target markets that are not interested in or in need of your offering is often detrimental to the overall effectiveness of the program. For example, spending by a local organization on national television advertising is highly inefficient and costly in terms of return. The same point applies to those seeking change in health, sport, and physical activity.

If carried out in an efficient manner that reaches key audiences in a relevant way, a communications strategy can have benefits beyond the conveying of information. Indeed, an organization's message can help attract more sponsorship and encourage people to raise funds and volunteer for the related cause. In the next chapters, we will explore those expanded benefits in detail. Specifically, we will examine how a communications plan relates to attracting more sponsor and donor support and how role models and champions can help drive marketing messages forward to desired groups and wider audiences than any partner might have imagined.

In summary, your message and marketing strategy must be based on your own resources and assets but also guided by the way that your target groups find and use information. Clearly, your communications strategy, like the partnership itself, is unique to you and your partner and to your partnership goals, visions, and objectives.

CHAPTER 4

The Value of Sponsorship in Physical Activity, Sport Participation, and Health

As outlined in chapter 3, a well-communicated and planned partnership can have considerable benefits beyond the core goals of the particular cause associated with the partnership. Further, those additional benefits can often add more value to the core effort through the resources that they can generate. This is the case with sponsorship, or perhaps more appropriately, corporate sponsorship. To illustrate, consider the case of the United States Olympic Committee (USOC). The USOC is the rights holder for the Olympic Games and the Olympic Rings in the United States. A charitable, not-for-profit organization, the USOC has a mandate to field the national team at the Olympic Games and Pan American Games, as well as support the high-performance, development, and grassroots elements of all Olympic and Pan American sports in the United States. In its activities to pursue its objectives, the USOC is involved in many elements of Olympics-related sport in the United States that are attractive to corporations that would like to associate with the images and values of the USOC and the Olympic Games, leverage the USOC's teams and events to reach relevant target markets, and incorporate athletes and teams into their marketing programs.

Because of the attractive platforms offered to corporations seeking to market their offerings and build their brands, sponsorship has grown dramatically over the past 30 years in North America, Europe, Asia, and Australia. More recently, as sponsorship has established itself as a marketing strategy for organizations and as competition for sponsors and the pursuit of properties (sponsees) who provide high value to sponsors has increased, sponsorship of not-for-profits and causes has grown considerably. As a form of partnership, sponsorship has become an important tool for organizations seeking to engage in public–private partnerships. This chapter presents, describes, and provides direction on sponsorship in the context of partnerships between corporate sponsors and not-for-profit organizations active in sport, health, and physical activity.

Sponsorship is a contemporary and growing marketing tactic that has been getting more attention and a greater proportion of marketing budgets despite constraints in marketing budgets in most sectors since 2008 (IEG 2011; Canadian Sponsorship Landscape Study 2011). Sponsorship has moved away from its philanthropic roots and today is largely viewed as part of marketing strategy in which organizations exchange promotional value for resources to achieve the goals of their respective organizations (Seguin and O'Reilly 2007). This transformation signals the effectiveness of sponsorship in reaching targets through cluttered marketplaces and intense competition. Although this book focuses on many forms of partnership, sponsorship is one of the most important given its demonstrated growth and effectiveness.

Tactically, a sponsorship takes place one when organization (the sponsor) provides cash or in-kind products or services to another organization (the sponsee) in exchange for opportunities to promote or activate their products, brands, or corporate reputation. Authors have described a sponsorship as "a strategic activity with the potential to generate a sustainable competitive advantage in the marketplace" (Fahy, Farrelly, and Quester 2004, p. 1013) or an arrangement in which a "corporation creates a link with an outside issue or event, hoping to influence the audience by the connection" (Rifon, Choi, Trimble, and Li 2004, p. 30). This association, or link, is what differentiates sponsorship from other marketing tactics and, most important for this book, enables corporate partners to borrow from the associations and goodwill attached to not-for-profit organizations in sport, health, and physical activity. By definition, engaging in a sponsorship with a not-for-profit partner (sponsee) allows the investor (sponsor) to receive related promotional benefits (e.g., media exposure) as well as the association with the images and attributes of the sponsee and the related cause, which has been shown to influence the affinity of participants to that cause (see Irwin, Lachowetz, Cornwell, and Clark 2003). In their research, Irwin et al. surveyed spectators at a professional golf tournament sponsored by Federal Express (FedEx) and partnered with a hospital. Results of their research at the 2000 FedEx St. Jude Classic Golf Tournament suggest that spectators' opinions of the sponsor (FedEx) were influenced in a positive manner through the association to the cause (i.e., St. Jude Children's Research Hospital).

Sponsorship is also known to sponsors for its ability to allow efficient reach to specific target markets (Pham and Johar 2001). This aspect is particularly relevant to health-related sponsees who often have a following with strong affinity (e.g., athletes supporting their sport, cancer survivors, affected family members). Despite these affinities, in today's competitive marketplace, sponsorship is not easy for most sponsees (except for elite properties such as the Olympic Games, FIFA World Cup, and the Super Bowl). Sponsees compete for limited sponsorship opportunities in an environment where the demand from sponsees for sponsorship resources is significantly greater than the supply of interested sponsors. Indeed, most sponsees seeking resources struggle to attract, satisfy, and maintain sponsors (Hoek and Gendall 2002). This challenge is even more significant in the sectors relevant to this book because these not-for-profits are often small and have limited resource bases, low levels of marketing expertise, and poor media coverage.

The following sections present three key topic areas in sponsorship (image transfer, stakeholders, and industry size) and their relevance to the sectors of interest to this book (sport participation, physical activity, and health).

Image Transfer

In sponsorships between corporations and not-for-profit sport, physical activity, and health organizations, transfer of images is a key element that attracts the interest of the private sector when they are making their marketing decisions. Image transfer is an integral conceptual element of understanding how sponsorship works. Much research has been undertaken related to image transfer in sponsorship. The consensus of those researchers is that both parties in a sponsorship bring their own image values to the partnership and, through the sponsorship association (i.e., the joint message communicated to audiences such as the CIBC Run for the Cure or the Gatorade Hawaii Ironman Triathlon), those images, if leveraged properly, can be transferred by consumer perceptions to each other to the benefit of both parties (Gwinner and Eaton 1999).

Specific to public–private partnerships involving sponsorship with health, sport, and physical activity sponsees, note that this transfer takes place in the minds of the target audiences who transfer, through the sponsor–sponsee association, some image value from one party to another (see Gierl and Kirchner 1999). Taking this sort of lens to sponsorship in these contexts reveals why sport, health, and physical activity sponsees are of interest to corporate partners, because the importance of transferring images such as charity, health, not-for-profit, cause, and youth to corporations, brands, and products has considerable advantages in positioning versus competitors. When the sponsor has images that are dissimilar or inconsistent with the sponsee (e.g., a soft drink manufacturer and a youth-focused physical activity organization), increased activation and responsible implementation of the partnership (see appendix B, *The Partnership Protocol*) are necessary because research has shown that the more similar the images are, the easier the transfer of images will be (Gwinner and Eaton 1999). Similarly, the more involved the sponsor becomes with the sponsee, the stronger the perceived relationship will be. In turn, the ability to transfer image will be enhanced. This speaks strongly to the strength of the partnership: The stronger the partnership is, the stronger the benefits are.

Stakeholders: Sponsors, Sponsees, and Agencies

When considering sponsorship as a potential source of revenue, managers and marketers from the not-for-profit health, sport, or physical activity not-for-profit need to understand the players, or stakeholders, involved in sponsorship with a private-sector partner. Although many organizations and individuals will be involved with a sponsorship, there are three key stakeholder groups.

In the sponsorships relevant to this book, the corporate sponsor (e.g., Coke, Pepsi, IBM) is a private for-profit corporation that invests resources in a not-for-profit sponsee. In return, the corporate sponsor seeks to fulfill marketing objectives from their association with that sponsee.

The sponsee of interest here, and second stakeholder group, is a not-for-profit organization whose purpose is related to sport participation, health, or physical activity. Examples include ParticipACTION, United Way, American Cancer Society, Big Brothers and Sisters, and Motivate Canada. In a sponsorship, these sponsees receive resources (either cash or in-kind product or service) and may seek to achieve their own marketing objectives from the association.

The final important stakeholder group includes all affiliated entities who act as intermediaries in support of the partnership between the sponsor and the sponsee. This group, known as agencies, includes a sponsorship sales agent or agency that sells sponsorship on behalf of the sponsee or a marketing agent working for the sponsor. In the case of sponsorships in sport participation, health behaviors, or physical activity, agencies can take on important roles in ensuring that a partnership is successful. For example, a market research agency could analyze the effectiveness of the sponsorship to aid the sponsee in renewing the partnership. Similarly, a not-for-profit organization with no in-house marketing expertise may engage an agent to help develop a plan to attract sponsorship.

Building Partners Through Charity Sponsorship

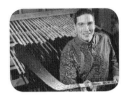

Aaron Logan

President, Heritage Stick Company

BIO

Aaron Logan is the president of Heritage Stick Co. He has worked in the hockey and golf industry for the past 14 years in sales, broadcasting, and management capacities. Heritage Stick Co. supplies branded sport-related products to teams, players, and special events as well as celebrity event management services. Aaron currently resides in Queensville, Ontario, with his wife, Melanie, and their two children.

MY VIEW ON PARTNERSHIPS

As an entrepreneur starting a new business, I had to look at every angle to help get my business off the ground. Working with charities and not-for-profits helped me grow my business while I help the charities build their brand within the community and achieve their fund-raising goals. About 15 to 20 percent of my business is working with charities including Right To Play, Cystic Fibrosis Canada, Team Up Foundation, and the Canadian Cancer Society. In the past six years, my partnerships have grown as I provide promotional hockey sticks for special events and foundations related to the NHL, AHL, CHL, and former players. Partnering with charities and foundations is not just about dollars and cents or making money. Instead, I see the partnerships as a way to make connections with people and organizations that might be interested in my product, while also getting to take part in something worthwhile. The events that I take part in have meaning to me; I want to be a part of them, and the charities want me there.

IMPORTANCE OF WORKING WITH CHARITIES

As an advisory board member of the Princess Margaret Hospital Foundation, I've been able to devote time to the Road Hockey to Conquer Cancer event. By taking part in this and other charity special events, I've been able to capture some media spotlight and gain recognition that has been good for my business. I don't go to events to sell, but the events are avenues to make contacts. In my business I don't sell directly to the public, but being part of a hockey charity event puts me in touch with other businesses and executives that might be interested in our products. The word of mouth that you can generate by taking part in special events is fantastic; you're able to showcase your management style and the way that you relate to teams and athletes.

Charities are changing; they have to align themselves with corporations and business to attract new fund-raising dollars. It gives people more comfort to see a trusted company associated with a charity when they are considering where to put their donation dollars. In other words, trust in a company builds more trust in the charity. Aligning with private partners translates into a more positive public perception of the charity.

(continued) ▶

(continued) ▶

CHAMPIONING CHARITIES: CELEBRITY PRESENCE

In bigger cities like Toronto (Canada), special events occur every day of the summer and are scheduled throughout the rest of the year. Many events use paid celebrities to help fund-raise and drive ticket sales for special events. In contrast, I was in a smaller city (Sudbury, Canada) this year for a charity event and was surprised by the lack of celebrity presence. Some charities seem to have an old way of thinking in that they should not pay for certain things, even things that can improve their events. The shifting reality that you see in more successful charities is that you have to spend money to make money. Expecting people to devote time and resources is a hard sell, especially the busy celebrities who seem to be a good fit for the charity. Many celebrities have a charity that is close to their hearts, so they will work with the charity at no cost. Some will volunteer for events or allow the charity to use their names and images. But the reality is that people are busy; athletes and celebrities are working and training 12 months a year and have to balance that with other family and personal commitments. Paying celebrities for their presence at a charity event may be a way for them to justify devoting their time. The practice is well accepted, and appearance fees range from $500 to over $10,000 depending on the celebrity and the event. Having a celebrity present at key charity events can boost fund-raising efforts and donations. I recently put hockey celebrity Darryl Sittler in a Rotary Club luncheon event in North Bay (Canada). The normal luncheon attendance was about 100 people, but with Darryl Sittler taking part, attendance exceeded 350 and much more money was raised. In this case, the appearance fee provided much more for the charity in return.

BUILDING RELATIONSHIPS

As a small business, you want to partner with people and charities that you believe in. For me, a partnership with an organization like the Team Up Foundation (part of Maple Leaf Sports and Entertainment) means more than just my supplying sticks and pucks; it's a way to help me build awareness about my company with the right people. My link to the foundation sets the groundwork for building relations with the Toronto Maple Leafs NHL team and other hockey-related organizations. You can always put in more than you get out, but when you are committed to the charity and to relationship building, then the returns will come. With the Kings Care Foundation, the charity of the L.A. Kings NHL team, I started the relationship by purchasing a package of tickets that I could donate back to the foundation; the result is that three years later the L.A. Kings are still buying sticks from me. As a small business, I appreciate the reciprocal cycle; I provide good customer service and products to an associated foundation, and that effort helps build my name in the organization.

ADVICE FOR BUILDING AND MAINTAINING PARTNERSHIPS

1. Align yourself with good partners that you believe in. Your heart has to be in it; choose a charity that affects your family or resonates with your interests.
2. Know your business future and where you want to grow.

3. You'll get tons of calls from charities, and you can't support them all; it's OK to say no.

4. If you are going to get involved, then go all in.

5. Time may be easier to give than money sometimes, but it can be just as valuable.

Don't just follow the big charities. You'll accomplish more with a charity that is the best fit for you and your business even if it's a smaller charity or event.

GLOBAL APPLICATION QUESTIONS

1. Why would Heritage Stick Company care about public–private partnerships?

2. As an entrepreneur, Logan has spent considerable time and energy working with and supporting charities. Why is this activity important for his businesses?

3. Logan discusses the idea that charities are changing. What three key points is he making?

Size and Scope of the Sponsorship Industry

As noted earlier in the chapter, sponsorship has grown rapidly in terms of its use and the amount that organizations are spending on rights fees. Estimates of the size of the industry have been made over the past 30 years, with varying accuracy. Today, two organizations measure the amount invested annually in sponsorship: IEG in the United States and globally and the Canadian Sponsorship Landscape Study (CSLS) in Canada.

In terms of global investment in sponsorship, studies have shown an increase from around US$500 million in 1982 to US$3 billion in 1989 to an estimated US$48.7 billion in 2011 (IEG 2011). In 2011 IEG estimated North American spending at US$18.2 billion. The CSLS has tracked sponsorship spending in Canada since 2006, when spending was estimated at CDN$1.11 billion, through to 2010, when the estimate hit CDN$1.55 billion (Canadian Sponsorship Landscape Study 2011).

Strategic Sponsorship

This section of chapter 4 builds on the first section but focuses specifically on corporate sponsorship in the sport, physical activity, and health sectors. It builds on the foundations of sponsorship as an effective, growing, and collaborative type of partnership. This section touches on four particularly important strategic elements of sponsorship: association, activation, exclusivity, and evaluation.

Association

The association between the sponsor and the sponsee, as noted earlier, is of the utmost importance in any sponsorship, but this importance is enhanced in corporate sponsorship of not-for-profits in health, sport, and physical activity for two key reasons. First, not-for-profit organizations in these sectors have the ability to provide their corporate-sector partners with highly positive and beneficial images that they, in turn, can activate around to achieve their own objectives. Second, because of their status as not-for-profit organizations, these health, sport, and physical activity organizations are under increased scrutiny from their members, the media, and other stakeholders in how they carry out their business and whom they partner with.

The importance of the association in the context topics of this book can be observed in public examples when medical associations partner with private-sector organizations with whom they have a disconnect (including soft drink manufacturers and food manufacturers). As described in *The Partnership Protocol* (see chapter 2), when this disconnect is considerable, the not-for-profit partner faces two realities: (*a*) An opportunity is present for increased generation of revenue through the partnership because of the enhanced benefit to the corporate partner, and (*b*) entering into such a partnership presents the risk of negative backlash from media, members, and other stakeholders.

Activation

One of the key elements of sponsorship is activation, or investment by the parties above and beyond the rights fees to promote the association, reach target markets, and increase the image transfer process. Activation, specifically used in the context of corporate sponsorship of not-for-profit organizations in health, sport, and physical activity, refers to strategies that the sponsor or sponsee funds in addition to what was outlined in the contract and then implements to increase the effectiveness of the sponsorship. These techniques are varied and could include such approaches as developing commercials for the sponsored property and paying for their diffusion leading up to, during, and following the event (Nicholls, Roslow, and Dublish 1999).

Several important points apply here for not-for-profits in health, sport, and physical activity. First, without activation, sponsorship is not effective, and other marketing tactics (e.g., advertising) would be better choices (Seguin and O'Reilly 2007). The take-away here for not-for-profits is that they must ensure that their corporate partner activates if they hope for a successful partnership and renewal or long-term continuation. Second, the ability to leverage a sponsorship extensively as part of an integrated marketing communications mix is one of the elements that make it more attractive than other promotional tools such as advertising and publicity (Cornwell, Pruitt, and Clark 2005). This aspect needs to be considered and communicated in the sales, renewal, and evaluation stages of a sponsorship.

Exclusivity

A vitally important strategic element of most sponsorships is exclusivity. The concept of exclusivity refers to a sponsor being given the right to be the only sponsor of a given event in their business category (e.g., automobile, airline, and so on). In many cases, exclusivity is known to be a key element of

Partnership Highlight

LOCAL TORONTO PARK RECEIVES EARLY HOLIDAY GIFT
FROM COCA-COLA CANADA AND PARTNERS

As part of its continued mandate of encouraging people to "Live Positively," Coca-Cola Canada—through a unique partnership between itself, ParticipACTION, Parks Canada, Toronto Community Housing, and Bienenstock Natural Playgrounds—will be undertaking a project to completely rejuvenate Moss Park in Toronto for spring 2012. The park, which in recent years had fallen into disrepair, will soon be home to a brand new soccer field, a large vegetable garden for residents to enjoy, and increased seating facilities.

"Through the Coca-Cola Foundation, we are proud to be investing $125,000 in this important project which will encourage more active living through the building of a sustainable natural playground," said Nicola Kettlitz, president of Coca-Cola Canada. "This project fits with our Live Positively commitment to make a positive contribution in the communities where we operate."

The other partners in this project—ParticipACTION, Bienenstock Natural Playgrounds, Parks Canada, and Toronto Community Housing—are all involved for multiple reasons, but the common goal of making a difference in the lives of residents through the Moss Park Rejuvenation project unites them all. The organizations involved hope that others will take note of the success of this multiple-partner project and will seek to engage in similar types of partnerships.

ParticipACTION's involvement with the project stems from the organization's position as the country's leading proponent of physical activity and sport participation.

"We are proud to be a part of this multisectoral collaboration to create a space where all residents can be active and connect with nature," says Kelly Murumets, president and CEO of ParticipACTION. "Research shows that children and youth who spend time outdoors are more physically active, which leads to improved health and well-being."

Bienenstock Natural Playgrounds sought input and feedback from residents during the entire design process. During the course of three months, over 1,400 residents of Moss Park were invited to attend meetings to voice what features they would like to see included in the new park.

"The Moss Park Rejuvenation project is an amazing opportunity to provide opportunities for youth to connect with nature in an urban setting," says Alan Latourelle, CEO, Parks Canada. "As part of this collaboration, we will be offering a hands-on immersive experience for youth to spend a couple of days at Georgian Bay Islands National Park to build a deeper and long-term connection with our natural and historic heritage."

"This is an exciting opportunity for Toronto Community Housing and our Moss Park residents," said Deborah Simon, COO of Toronto Community Housing. "Aside from hours of active fun for children of all ages, this partnership will also help build a safe and healthy community by reclaiming the outdoor space around the buildings."

GLOBAL APPLICATION QUESTIONS

1. This partnership example highlights a number of key elements about multiparty (more than two) partnerships. List three of these and explain each.
2. From a business perspective, why do you think that Bienenstock Natural Playgrounds is part of this partnership?
3. From a government perspective, why do you think that Parks Canada is part of this partnership?

successful sponsorship, and it is often given credit for creating the high level of interest in sponsoring the Olympic Movement in the mid-1980s (Pound 1996). This success stems from the fact that exclusivity reduces, if not removes, the influence of ambush marketing by the sponsor's competitors, who seek to create confusion in consumers or target audiences as to whom the official sponsor is. Exclusivity is important to sponsors because some proportion of audiences support organizations that are the official sponsors of causes or properties that they believe in or support (O'Reilly et al. 2008).

In practice, exclusivity, or category exclusivity as it is now often termed, is becoming increasingly important. Studies of consumer opinion of ambush marketing (Seguin, Lyberger, O'Reilly, and McCarthy 2005) demonstrate empirically that consumers find ambush marketing unacceptable and are confused by it, making exclusivity key to success in sponsorship with large properties, although less so with smaller properties. For the vast majority of sponsees in the contexts topical to this book, rendering exclusivity may therefore be less important with respect to the overall impact of the sponsorship. But it is not the overall impact that matters; it is the interest of the potential (or current) corporate partner in exclusivity that the not-for-profit must keep in mind. As such, it is recommended that the not-for-profit work to guarantee exclusivity in these partnerships.

Evaluation

The final key strategic element for both parties to consider, particularly the not-for-profit partner, is sponsorship evaluation. The evaluation of sponsorship is a much-discussed area of need in both sponsorship research and practice (O'Reilly and Madill 2009). Both IEG (2011) and the Canadian Sponsorship Landscape Study (2011) reveal that investments in evaluation of sponsorship are low and suggest that much more is needed industry-wide.

The need for an improved approach to sponsorship evaluation (Crompton 2004) is based on four drivers: (a) that current practice is largely proprietary and not shared, (b) that advocates for sponsorship need empirical proof of its effectiveness, (c) that not-for-profit sponsees need evidence to negotiate for new sponsors and renewal with current sponsors, and (d) that intermediaries (e.g., marketing agencies, media partners, cosponsors, and others who assist in the establishment and maintenance of sponsorships) whose role it is to broker sponsorship contracts between sponsors and sponsees need improved evaluation to develop, negotiate, and finalize sponsorship contracts.

Finding a Sponsor for Your Not-for-Profit

If you are reading this book as a representative, employee, or board member of a not-for-profit organization seeking to improve its partnerships or begin developing new partners, this section is highly relevant to you. In pulling from the previous sections and adding some of our experiences, we provide a series of steps to follow to determine whether finding a sponsor makes sense for your not-for-profit and, if so, what steps should be implemented to maximize the benefits of this arrangement. The process includes 10 steps, as detailed in table 4.1.

TABLE 4.1　10 Steps in Finding a Sponsor for Your Not-for-Profit

Step	Objective	Prospective sponsee action
1	Determine mutual interests	Determine whether the potential sponsor shares a common interest with you or a shared goal to achieve the cause or benefit of interest to the partnership.
2	Identify and communicate partnership goals to the prospective sponsor	Determine whether the potential sponsor realizes and understands your goals and the goals of the partnership, including the relevant health, physical activity, wellness, or fitness goals.
3	Research and profile prospective partners	Undertake diligent market research to develop a profile of potential partners. Then review these profiles internally.
4	Determine the desired longevity of the partnership	Review documents and talk, where appropriate, to the client to ascertain whether the potential sponsor offers opportunities for a successful, long-term partnership.
5	Understand the potential for sharing resources	Forecast the expertise, resources, reach, and assets that the prospective sponsor could bring to the sponsorship and to your organization.
6	Assess your organization's ability to commit time and energy	Assess the sponsorship opportunity by considering the alternative activities that could be undertaken with the time and resources that your organization will be required to invest in the sponsorship (as determined in step 5).
7	Find champions	Appoint a supported individual at each of the organizations involved to act as a champion for the prospective sponsorship—one at the sponsor (private sector) and one at the sponsee (public sector). These individuals will make sure that high-level dialogue and commitment to the partnership's objectives occur.
8	Determine mutual participant or target group and stakeholder benefits	Carry out research that reviews the potential sponsor's current and sought target audiences and the way in which these match with your stakeholders. The objective is to identify common targets that could be of benefit to both.
9	Assess risk	Assess and evaluate the relative risks and rewards of entering into the sponsorship. For example, consider the overall brand of the proposed sponsorship in the context of the brands of each organization involved (i.e., sponsor, sponsee, agency). A second example would be an assessment of both parties' capacity to fulfill partnership promises. Do you both have the will and the means to deliver? Do partners share accountability and responsibility for partnership outcomes?
10	Determine disconnects and ways to manage them	Search for disconnects (i.e., products, services, or brand elements that have considerable opposite meaning to your brand, products, and services). After identifying those elements, set policy direction for each disconnect based on a decision by the board using the criteria to consider potential partners in certain sponsorship categories.

Motivation and Mutual Respect in Partnership Building

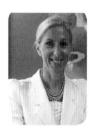

Bev Deeth

President and CEO, Concerned Children's Advertisers (CCA)

BIO

Bev Deeth is the president of Concerned Children's Advertisers (CCA). She is responsible for the strategic direction of the organization and works to set the national standard for due diligence in the social-marketing area. CCA is a unique not-for-profit organization and model of corporate social responsibility. Made up of 17 Canadian member companies and supported by numerous partners, including child-centered advertisers, broadcasters, and issue experts, CCA is committed to understanding and contributing solutions to issues of challenge in children's lives. As committed Canadian advertisers, CCA has the mission of being the credible, caring, and authoritative voice of responsible children's advertising and communications. The organization provides resources for and has expertise in reaching and teaching Canadian kids about how to deal effectively with the issues that challenge their daily lives. Mrs. Deeth has more than 15 years of senior management experience in the community development, philanthropy, health care, and sport sectors.

VIEW ON PARTNERSHIPS

I have a very positive view of partnerships. Every sector should be considered as your organization goes through the prospecting stage. In my world most partnerships are multisectorial and not limiting of one partner or another. This combination can be powerful. Think of academia, government, corporations, not-for-profits, and so on, depending on the issue and task at hand. All bring a different lens and a different advantage to the table. We need to understand that by working together our perspectives are much stronger and more powerful than when we work in isolation. Working in partnerships, however, is not without challenges. A key ingredient to any successful partnership is mutual respect and trust, as well as a clear understanding of each other's business objectives, goals, and corporate values.

PARTNERSHIPS AS A SOURCE OF ORGANIZATIONAL MOTIVATION

I have extensive experience in the not-for-profit, fund-raising, and partnerships worlds, and I want to begin my contribution to this book by stressing that there is nothing more rewarding than securing a long-term, lucrative, and productive partnership. Your entire organization will benefit at all levels from having a new, strong corporate partner, and the partnership will provide all stakeholders with a renewed sense of credibility and excitement. It is the fuel that keeps us fund-raisers going!

PARTNERSHIP BENEFITS ARE BROADER THAN WE THINK

Partnerships between for-profit and not-for-profit organizations are interesting. The whole concept is often based on financial exchanges; therefore, we often forget about the other nonfinancial pieces that for-profits can bring to the table, and these benefits are substantial. In our case—at CCA—we receive other nonfinancial support from our many corporate partners including intellectual resources (i.e., advice, committee participation, expertise, knowledge sharing, and so on) and marketing muscle (i.e., media assets, networks, marketing resources, connection to other partners, and so on), as well as pro bono contributions from these partners. I can't stress enough how important these considerations are.

As an example, at CCA our broadcast members (CTV, Shaw Media, Teletoon, CBC, and Corus) donate pro bono airtime in excess of $4.3 million in 2010. This provides us with great reach nationally to all our audiences and allows us to invest in the production and creation of innovative social marketing campaigns. They see great value in our work and are proud to showcase our messages to their key audiences.

WHAT IS IN IT FOR ME?

Many not-for-profits come with their hands out asking for donations or swag from corporations with nothing to offer in return. Those days are gone, and today's partnerships are measured by value. Return on investment (ROI) is measured now more than ever before. We need to work toward a healthy, productive, sharing, and win–win relationship that is dynamic, continues to grow, deals with issues and programs together, and lasts a long time.

MUTUAL RESPECT IN PARTNERSHIPS

I am a big believer in relationship building. In the business environment you encounter a multitude of personalities. This is where enhanced people skills, reputation, and the development of positive relationships come into play. Specific elements of any relationship are based on the personalities involved and must be oriented toward building mutual trust. Both sides need to be open minded, able to see opportunities that exist, able to understand their partner's perspective, and do things in a respectful way.

I personally know a number of managers from corporations who invest in our field—the prevention of childhood obesity—who might not be viewed positively by some, but who have helped in significant ways because they are open to opportunities, change, communication, and considering ways to work together toward the cause. Never underestimate the power of face-to-face interaction.

We all have our own business objectives, and when we develop a partnership with anybody, we all have our own priorities. At the end of the day, we want to achieve these. So, all parties need to go in with an open mind and undertake the appropriate due diligence to explore the objectives of the partner or potential partner. Don't be afraid to dip your toe in the water and take a risk. Realize that things change—the environment, specific organizations involved, and the causes of interest.

(continued) ▶

(continued) ▶

If you look at our organization model at CCA, we've had a core funding model from a number of member companies for the past 21 years, many of them for the entire time. Although our cause focus has changed over time, the companies have been with us despite these changes. They are aligned by their belief in our core principles and see great value in our work. So, it is interesting that we are now being challenged on having these partners because our current main issue is childhood obesity. But they have supported us long before that became an issue of importance. CCA has a 21-year reputation of reaching and teaching Canadian children, and it is this underlying objective that binds these companies in this unique and successful model. I applaud them for their passion and support of our cause.

CRISIS MANAGEMENT IN PARTNERSHIPS

When you align with a brand, you take on risks that may be linked to that brand in the future. You must have those tough conversations at the onset and thoroughly talk through a crisis management plan. Partnerships today are much more risky than they were years ago. Reputation and credibility are important, and we, as a not-for-profit, must protect ourselves.

CAUSE MARKETING 101

A number of great examples are out there to consider when looking at a cause marketing campaign to drive fund-raising efforts. Immediately, CIBC's Run for the Cure comes to mind as a best-in-class example because when I hear the name, I immediately associate it with cancer. So, I define this as best in class because they've done a great job with brand recognition and the association of that brand to the national cause and raising millions of dollars. It is simply Cause Marketing 101.

ADVICE FOR MANAGERS IN NOT-FOR-PROFIT ORGANIZATIONS SEEKING CORPORATE PARTNERSHIPS

I'd suggest a few specific things:

1. Make sure to do your research and prospecting up front. This is probably the most critical thing that you can do. Find organizations that have a reason, a rationale, or an impetus to get involved with you.

2. Manage your organization like a brand—develop unique selling properties (USPs).

3. Use your board of directors to make introductions and open doors. Recruit board members who have both affluence, the ability to make a contribution, and influence, the ability to attract others to make contributions. Influential people will attract other influential people. Strong volunteer leadership will define your organization.

4. Understand that large corporations get an overwhelming number of calls for support and that they listen only to those who have a very good fit and well-articulated partnership plan. You get only one chance, so make it good!

5. Cultivate the partnership after it is signed by getting to know who the partner is and what their objectives are. Invest in recognizing the partners and their key employees, service them, grow the relationship, activate around the partnerships, and evaluate. This process is critical and ongoing.

6. Continue to look at value-added benefits during the term of the partnership because renewal is not always guaranteed.

GLOBAL APPLICATION QUESTIONS

1. Deeth, who leads Concerned Children's Advertisers, has "a very positive view of partnerships." Why?

2. Deeth emphasizes trust in partnerships. Why is this important?

3. Name two key benefits of partnerships that Deeth says are broader than we think in terms of their effect.

Profile of a Sponsee

What is a sponsee? Often called a property by practitioners working in sponsorship, the sponsee is a relatively complex entity in sponsorship. This complexity stems largely from the fact that many more properties are interested in becoming sponsees than there are available resources from sponsors for sponsorship. With the exception of what we call megasponsees (i.e., major properties with vast reach and marketing value like the Olympic Games, Super Bowl, Academy Awards, World's Fair, Cannes Film Festival, and FIFA World Cup), most properties, or typical sponsees, have to compete amongst themselves to find, sign, and retain sponsors. This take-away is important for not-for-profit organizations in health, sport participation, and physical activity that are typically not the most attractive property for sponsors to partner with in terms of pure marketing benefit (i.e., reach, access to target markets, ability to access national and international media) when compared with professional sport, the arts, and festivals. Indeed, it is the link to a cause and a benefit that even allows health and physical activity properties to be in the choice set for sponsors.

The Canadian Sponsorship Landscape Study provides us with some good data on who sponsees are in Canada (which is likely to be similar to the landscape of sponsees in most developed countries). The 2011 version of the study was the fifth annual version, in which 218 sponsees (organizations who receive sponsorship resources from sponsors) responded to the survey (CSLS 2011). The sample respondents included sponsees whose reach was primarily international (15.1 percent), national (30.3 percent), provincial or multiprovincial (27.7 percent), regional (12.6 percent), and local or municipal (14.3 percent). The CSLS (2011) also provided a general profile of sponsees, which revealed that the average annual budget was $5,358,179; the average sponsorship revenue for a sponsee was $1,896,864 (a 3.1 percent increase over 2009);

the average staff size was 390 paid employees, 5 of whom worked directly on sponsorship; and the average volunteer team size was 752 volunteers, 39 of whom worked on sponsorship. In terms of sponsee type, the CSLS (2011) sample was composed of festivals, fairs, and annual events (14.6 percent); sport (33.8 percent); entertainment, tours, and attractions (2.3 percent); arts (8.5 percent); cause (20.0 percent); and other (20.8 percent, including such things as facilities, education, museums, local and municipal governments, universities, and so on). According to the CSLS (2011), not-for-profit sponsees accounted for 83.7 percent of sponsees in the study. The average amount of cash sponsorship that a not-for-profit sponsee received annually was $1.45 million, with an average of $37,292 per sponsorship. The balance, for-profit sponsees, received 15.6 percent of rights fees from sponsors, an average of $3.06 million annually in cash sponsorship, with an average size of each individual sponsorship estimated to be $66,448 (CSLS 2011).

Finding a Not-for-Profit Sponsee for Your For-Profit Corporation

Those who work in the not-for-profit health, physical activity, and sport participation sectors need to realize that selling sponsorship is not easy. In fact, it is difficult. With the exception of megaevents that have vast television audiences and reach, most organizations struggle to compete for scarce corporate-sector resources. Despite the fact that sponsorship is growing—now estimated to be CDN$1.55 billion in Canada (CSLS 2011) and US$17.2 billion in North America (IEG 2011)—competition for sponsorship is growing faster (CSLS 2011), and global sport, arts, and festival properties are taking large proportions of available money. Coupled with streamlined government spending and increasing numbers of small not-for-profits, this circumstance renders sponsorship sales challenging for small not-for-profits working in health, sport participation, and physical activity.

One of the best sources of learning how to compete in sponsorship as a small property is to learn from those who have done well in achieving sponsorship in similar situations. Here, we introduce the case study of the 2011 Garnier FindingLife Expedition to Africa. In this case, a small, youth-focused, social-media-based not-for-profit, FindingLife, partnered with a corporate sponsor, Garnier, on an integrated sponsorship that was activated considerably by both parties. For the sponsor, one of their staff was identified and took part in the expedition, which included a three-phase (mountain climb, school build, safari) adventure over three weeks in a poor part of Kenya, Africa (an area known as Solio). The adventure included 6 high school students each from both Canada and Kenya (12 total), who were identified by FindingLife following a social media competition linked to local schools. Throughout the expedition, media (film, web, and print) were generated around a number of themes, namely the youth involved, a charity Canada versus Kenya soccer game, internal webisodes prepared exclusively for the sponsor, and ongoing communication back to Canada from the team in each phase, including the summit day on the mountain. The process of finding the sponsor took the expedition leaders from FindingLife many months and many pitches. Key steps in the process involved providing media value back to sponsors, building a relationship with key members in the sponsor's organization, involving youth, including filmmaking and social media webisodes, and developing a competitive and active program to identify the participants.

Profile of a Sponsor

To profile a sponsor, we again draw on the fifth annual Canadian Sponsorship Landscape Study. The results for sponsors were based on a sample of 116 sponsor respondents. They had a median full-time staff of 500 (range of 10 to 35,000), mean annual sales of $415 million, and an average of about 100 sponsorships. Many (34.3 percent) had a national scope. They invested on average 22.3 percent of their overall marketing and communications budgets in sponsorship (CSLS 2011). The respondent sponsors came from all industry categories, and most (69.2 percent) invested in fewer than 50 sponsorships, although about 20 percent had 150 sponsorships or more (CSLS 2011).

Conclusion

Chapter 4 is about sponsorship. It outlines sponsorship as a growing and effective tactic used by marketers to achieve their promotional objectives. Investments in sponsorship rights is now estimated to be near US$50 billion globally and approaching US$20 million in North America. Many suggest that activation spending (i.e., additional spending to maximize the benefits of the sponsorship) amounts to that much again, more than doubling this investment. As such, sponsorship is a key type of partnership and one that we've positioned in our partnership continuum as an important phase in partnerships as organizations strive for collaborative, long-term relationships. Sponsorship is an element in the promotional mix of organizations—a business tactic that seeks to achieve business outcomes. Akin to our view that a partnership between a for-profit and not-for-profit organization in physical activity, sport participation, or public health is not philanthropy, rather, sponsorship is a decision with business outcomes, including cause-related marketing ones.

Sponsorship of a not-for-profit property is often associated with the sport sector, particularly the Olympic Games and megaevents like the FIFA World Cup, the IAAF World Athletics Championships, and other international and national events such as FINA World Aquatics Championships, the United States Olympic Trials, and others. As noted in the chapter, however, investments in sponsorship, although growing, have been diversifying in their targets. More money is going to festivals, entertainment, causes, and arts properties. This demonstration of corporate sponsors' interest in finding sponsorship partners (properties) who provide them with opportunities to achieve their objectives and to access their current and potential customers is highly relevant to partnerships with the not-for-profit sector. Not-for-profit organizations must recognize the need to (a) consider these relationships as two directional, (b) build strong relationships with partners and deliver on commitments made to those partners, and (c) always follow the tenets of *The Partnership Protocol*.

CHAPTER 5

Revenue Strategies for Not-for-Profit Organizations

Although private-sector partnerships are essential to the revenue strategies of many not-for-profit organizations, keep in mind that corporate fund-raising makes up a minority of overall not-for-profit sector revenues. In Canada, for example, of all sport and recreation organizations, corporate support made up only 15 percent of their overall revenues (Hall et al. 2005). Although this figure is five times higher than the average percentage of revenue provided by corporate support for not-for-profits, it is much smaller than the percentage of their revenue derived from fees for services provided and from membership fees. This chapter discusses the overall revenue streams of not-for-profits and highlights both the unique contributions of private–public partnerships to not-for-profits as well as other important revenue streams for organizations working in this sector. In this chapter we discuss many of the major funding streams for not-for-profit organizations including funds from government, fees for goods and services, and philanthropy, including corporate support, individual support, and support from foundations.

Data on Sport and Recreation Organizations

More than 100,000 sport and recreation organizations operate in the United States. These entities take in almost US$30 billion in revenue (National Center for Charitable Statistics 2011). For statistical purposes, sport and recreation organizations are classified according to the definition provided by Hall et al. (2005, p. 60); accordingly, the term *sports* includes "amateur sport, training, physical fitness and sport competition services and events. Includes fitness and wellness centers." Recreation and social clubs include "recreational facilities and services to individuals and communities. Includes playground associations, country clubs, men's and women's clubs, touring clubs and leisure clubs." Service organizations include "membership organizations providing services to members and local communities, such as Lions, Zonta International, Rotary and Kiwanis."

About 7 percent of U.S. not-for-profit organizations are involved with sport and recreation, and many more are registered with the IRS as social clubs. The entire not-for-profit sector in the United States had US$1.92 trillion in revenue in 2008, which at first glance makes sport and recreation organizations look like an almost insignificant part of the American not-for-profit sector. Official statistics, however, examine only organizations that are specifically focused on sport and recreation. The YMCA of Greater New York, which does considerable work in the field of sport and recreation and promoting healthy behavior, had revenues of $282 million in 2010 (YMCA of Greater New York 2011), but it would not be included in those statistics. Similarly, an after-school children's club that operated sport and recreation programs for at-risk kids would typically be considered a social services organization rather than a sport and recreation organization. In Canada, sport and recreation organizations

---

Steven Ayer, President of Common Good Strategies, is coauthor of Chapter 5.

are the most common type of not-for-profit, making up more than 30,000 of Canada's 160,000 not-for-profit organizations (Hall et al. 2005). Although sport and recreation organizations make up more than 20 percent of organizations, they tend to be considerably smaller than the average not-for-profit and took in only 5.5 percent of the total revenues of the Canadian not-for-profit sector, or slightly more than CDN$6 billion of the approximately CDN$125 billion in total revenues for not-for-profit organizations in Canada in 2003 (Hall et al. 2005). To further contextualize the relatively small size of sport and recreation organizations, consider that the annual revenue of sport and recreation organizations in Canada was slightly more than CDN$180,000, the lowest of more than 10 categories of not-for-profits examined (Hall et al. 2005). In contrast, in the same year, the average revenue for all not-for-profits in Canada was more than CDN$690,000, almost four times as much. Correspondingly, sport and recreation not-for-profits are more likely than any other category of organization to have no full-time staff. As mentioned earlier, however, many larger organizations that could be considered sport and recreation organizations, such as YMCAs and after-school clubs, are often classified in other categories, so their larger sizes would not be included in these statistics.

Government Sources

Sport and recreation organizations are quite different from many other types of not-for-profits in regard to the level of support that they receive from government. In Canada, although the typical not-for-profit receives about half of its revenues from governmental sources, at either the federal, provincial, or municipal level and through either direct grants or payment for services, sport and recreation organizations receive barely 10 percent of their total revenues from government sources (Hall et al. 2005). More than half of the total funding from government comes from the provincial level in Canada. Municipal governments provide almost 3 percent of total revenues for sport and recreation not-for-profits, which is higher than the average of only 1 percent. Despite the fact that many organizations note decreased government support, over the last 10 years total revenue from all levels of government has more than doubled in Canada (Charities Directorate 2010). In the United States, concrete statistics on the percentage of government revenue that goes to sport and recreation organizations is more difficult to obtain. Overall, however, only 8 percent of total revenue for U.S. public charities comes from government grants, and only 24 percent of total revenue comes from fees for services and goods from government (Wing, Roeger, and Pollak 2011). Given how much smaller total government support is for U.S. organizations (one-third of total revenues versus one-half of total revenues for Canadian not-for-profits), it is unlikely that the situation is any better for sport and recreation organizations looking for government support in the United States.

In general, government contributions to the not-for-profit sector usually take one of three forms: grants, contributions, and contracts (Scott 2003).

Grants, which are transfer payments to organizations, are subject to fewer rules about how the money should be spent. Contributions are similar to grants but tend to be more conditional about spending the money on a specific type of work. Contracts are specific agreements between the government and the not-for-profit to perform a specific service or provide a good. Typically, outputs and performance requirements are much clearer and more concrete in this case.

For sport and recreation organizations, infrastructure funding from government can be essential for completing projects that they would never otherwise be able to achieve. Even with for-profit organizations like a National Hockey League team, partnerships with local municipalities can be imperative for success, as outlined in the Executive Perspective of Kevin Compton (see chapter 7), cofounder of Radar Partners and co-owner of the NHL's San Jose Sharks. The city of San Jose owns the building and for 18 years has worked with the Sharks to ensure a mutually profitable relationship.

Government funding poses unique challenges despite some notable successes for organizations in the sport and recreation field. Among the challenging aspects of dealing with governments are the following (Hall et al. 2003):

- Delays in receiving funds
- Inconsistent reporting and compliance requirements
- Difficulty in receiving funding before expenses are incurred
- Constantly changing government rules and regulations
- High audit costs
- Constantly changing priorities
- Lack of coordination between government programs and funding priorities
- Being forced to change or eliminate programs based on changing government funding priorities

Fees for Goods and Services

The largest single source of revenues for sport and recreation tends to be fees for goods and services, either as a direct payment or through membership fees with the organization, typically from individuals though occasionally from organizations as well (Hall et al. 2005). Over time, a marked shift has occurred in that a greater proportion of all not-for-profit revenues are coming from this source, especially because governments are providing fewer grants or contributions and are entering into more contracts with not-for-profits (Dart and Zimmerman 2000; Scott 2003). This trend has not necessarily been good for not-for-profit organizations. Some have pointed out that contracts reduce an organization's autonomy and ability to adapt to changing environments (Salamon 1995). Because the not-for-profit has less ability to perform activities outside the contract (Dart and Zimmerman 2000), they cannot invest in strategic planning, evaluation, or basic infrastructure improvement that could produce superior results. Contracts may also have relatively low margins, which mean that it is difficult to increase overall organizational capacity. Although no specific statistics are available about the percentage of revenue that sport and recreation organizations receive from fees for goods and services in the United States, the overall not-for-profit sector receives 45.5 percent of its revenue from fees for services and goods from private sources, in addition to the 24.3 percent of total revenue coming from fees for services and goods from government (Wing, Roeger, and Pollak 2011). In Canada fees for goods and services from individuals made up 31 percent of the total revenues of sport and recreation organizations. An additional 25 percent of revenue was received from membership fees, and 7 percent came from charitable gaming fees. Charitable gaming fees have been declining in recent years (Scott 2003), particularly from bingo halls (Charities Directorate 2010).

Philanthropic Sources

Although many people assume that private philanthropy makes up a majority of not-for-profit sector revenue, in reality in both Canada and the United States fund-raising and philanthropic contributions make up only about 13 percent of total revenues (Hall et al. 2005; Wing, Roeger, and Pollak 2011).

Donations

Giving USA estimated that Americans gave US$212 billion in 2010 and an additional US$23 billion in bequests (Giving USA Foundation 2011). In Canada donations from individuals were estimated at only CDN$10 billion, a fraction of the total value of donations from individuals in the United States both in aggregate dollar value and in terms of donations per person. In Canada, with its much higher tax rates, a considerably higher portion of total sector revenues is provided by government and a much smaller portion by individuals (compare Hall et al. 2005 with Wing, Roeger, and Pollak 2010).

Unfortunately, none of the major sources for philanthropic data in the United States specifically examines sport and recreation organizations. In Canada, however, sport and recreation organizations received only 2 percent of the total value of donations (Hall et al. 2009), and 14 percent of Canadians donated to sport and recreation organizations. Of all 10 types of not-for-profits examined in both 2004 and 2007, sport and recreation organizations had the lowest average donation per person.

Overall, the top 10 percent of donors in Canada contributed more than 60 percent of overall donations (Hall et al. 2009). Even so, 84 percent of Canadians donated to an average of 3.8 charities and made an average annual gift of $437. The most common methods identified of donating to not-for-profits were mail requests, at shopping centers or on the street, door-to-door canvassing, church collections, sponsoring someone, charity events, in memoriam, and at work (Hall et al. 2009).

So, why do people give and what can not-for-profit organizations do to get more revenue from these donors? The most comprehensive review of motivations for donations was conducted by Bekkers and Wiepking (2010), who reviewed more than 500 scholarly articles and identified eight core reasons why people donate to charities:

1. Awareness of need
2. Solicitation
3. Costs and benefits
4. Altruism
5. Reputation
6. Psychological benefits
7. Values
8. Efficacy

After the fact, the eight motivations for giving almost seem simplistic, but careful study of each of these points can significantly improve an organization's ability to obtain donations. Essentially, potential donors need to be aware of a problem and be asked in some concrete way to give funds. They will weigh the personal costs of giving, including any potential tax benefits to reduce costs of giving. They may give out of altruism, they may give to improve their reputation, and they may give because it fits their values. Maybe their parents gave regularly when they were growing up and that is now part of how they view themselves. Some donors just give because of the great feelings they get from knowing that their contributions help people. Finally, an important consideration for many donors is whether their gift makes a difference. As with many topics in this book, evaluation or demonstration of impact is essential for donors and supporters of every kind, whether it's a private partner looking to contribute to a not-for-profit, a government donor, or an individual donor.

Each person will have these motivations weigh in on the donation decision to a different extent. The challenging part about this is understanding the individual donor and customizing strategies to facilitate donations that are specifically of interest to that donor. For example, many countries have numerous tax incentives to reduce the costs of giving. Although a donor is unlikely to give solely for tax purposes, organizations like the Partnership for Philanthropic Planning or the Canadian Association of Gift Planners, which have many members involved with major-gift fund-raising at charities, help ensure that their members are able to give advice to potential donors that may increase the size of the gift. Alternatively, looking at solicitations, multiple studies have found that more than 85 percent of donations are made within a few weeks of a solicitation by a not-for-profit. On the other hand, two of the biggest reasons that donors cite for failing to give more is that they receive too many solicitations and that they are unhappy with the methods of solicitations (Hall et al. 2009). Balancing these contrasting motivations and barriers to giving and striking the delicate balance in targeting donors properly goes a long way to maximizing potential donations.

In the spirit of partnerships that this book is focused on, potential partnerships should be examined in light of these eight motivations for supporting an organization. For example, how could a partnership with a corporation make individual donations more appealing? Many smaller charities have tremendous success when partnering with large organizations that can expose them to new donor audiences that they would never have the budget to reach. Alternatively, many corporations offer incentives for their employees to donate to causes, including making matching grants for employee gifts to particular charities (Ayer 2010). A relatively small initial gift can become much larger by leveraging these other channels of giving. Finally, with most effective partnerships, the partnership allows the not-for-profit to achieve goals that they would never be able to achieve without the partnership, which demonstrates to potential donors the importance of supporting the not-for-profit.

Foundations

A foundation is a particular type of charity that is created to give money to other types of charities. Generally, foundations give money only to charities and not to not-for-profits that are not registered charities, although there are some exceptions. The Foundation Center divides foundations into three different types—independent foundations, community foundations focused on particular geographic communities, and corporate foundations. In 2010 the Foundation Center estimated that foundations gave just under US$46 billion in total, down 2 percent from 2009 (Lawrence and Mukai 2011). Even so, the 2010 figure is a substantial increase from the estimated US$27.5 billion given in 2000.

Sport and recreation organizations are estimated to have received about 1.3 percent of total gifts in 2009 from foundations (Foundation Center 2011). Despite the relatively small percentage that sport and recreation organizations receive through this source, this book describes many instances of foundations that have significant partnerships involving work with sport and recreation. Examples include the RBC Foundation (a corporate foundation), which gave $100,000 in funding to increase access to cricket facilities, and the McConnell Foundation (an independent family foundation), which gave more than $1 million to True Sport to help reduce barriers to youth participation in hockey and soccer. Organizations involved in public or general health generally are more appealing to foundations and receive about 7 percent of foundation grants.

Independent foundations were estimated to give US$32.5 billion; corporate foundations, US$4.7 billion; and community foundations, US$4.1 billion. In the

United States there are slightly more than 76,000 grant-making foundations. A grant-making foundation is one that gives grants to other charities. Some foundations have decided instead to operate their own charitable programs and do not give grants to other charities (Lawrence and Mukai 2011). Canada has slightly more than 3,000 grant-making foundations (Hurvid, Ayer, and Ellison 2011). Although the recession decreased total foundation assets by 17 percent, overall giving by foundations in the United States fell by only 2.1 percent, which was still a record drop. In Canada foundations grew at almost four times the rate of other charities from 2000 to 2009 (Hurvid, Ayer, and Ellison 2011). Assets of Canadian foundations increased 75 percent between 2003 and 2008, although expenditures, while increasing rapidly, did not increase at quite that rate (Hurvid, Ayer, and Ellison 2011).

Hurvid, Ayer, and Ellison (2011) identified a few major reasons to consider using foundation fund-raising as part of your fund-raising strategy.

- Foundations are one of the fastest growing types of charities; there are more now than ever before.
- Foundation funding is one of the fastest growing sources of revenues for charities.
- Foundations can be an essential knowledge base for community organizations.
- Many foundations support the same partners for many years.
- Foundations can help an organization diversify its funding sources.

In the United States tools like the *Foundation Directory Online* provided by the Foundation Center (a national U.S. charity whose mission is to strengthen the social sector by advancing knowledge about philanthropy in the United States and around the world) can be used to find foundations specifically interested in funding a particular cause. In Canada the *Canadian Directory to Foundations & Corporations*, provided by Imagine Canada (a national Canadian charity dedicated to providing support for the charitable sector), serves a similar role. So, if you are looking for a particular foundation that may be interested in funding soccer in Iowa or helping you provide your after-school sport program for at-risk youth in Ottawa, Ontario, these tools can help.

Corporate Support

Using U.S. corporate tax returns, Giving USA estimates that U.S. corporates gave US$15.3 billion in cash contributions to not-for-profit organizations in 2010, an increase of more than 10 percent since 2009 and more than 23 percent since 2008 (Giving USA Foundation 2011). These statistics, however, likely underestimate to a significant degree the full amount of corporate support for not-for-profits (Ayer 2011). For example, in 2003 in Canada, tax-receipted donations by corporations amounted to CDN$1.3 billion. In the same year, a large-scale study of not-for-profits estimated total corporate support from donations and sponsorships at CDN$2.8 billion, more than double the amount reported on tax filings (Easwaramoorthy et al. 2006). Further, in 2003, 3 percent of Canadian corporations reported donating to charities on their tax returns, and representative surveys of Canadian businesses indicated that 78 percent of corporations made a donation (Ayer 2010), a massive difference. Typically, the largest donors report their donations on their tax returns, but small donors, which in aggregate are worth many billions of dollars in North America, are not captured by traditional methods of measuring corporate giving.

A major challenge with corporate support is that it tends to be concentrated among larger organizations. Representatives from smaller organizations and communities and less popular causes often complain that they are relatively cut off from this type of funding (Hall et al. 2003). Overall, a full 84 percent of corporate donations are made to the fewer than 1 in 10 not-for-profits that have more than $1 million in revenues (Easwaramoorthy et al. 2006). Smaller organizations can still receive support from corporations, both large and small, but seeking such support can be challenging (Ayer 2011). Note that donations of cash are but one of many ways that corporations support not-for-profit organizations. Many organizations of all sizes facilitate employee volunteering, sponsorships, cause-related marketing, donations of products, purchasing products or services from not-for-profits (including membership fees paid on behalf of employees), donations of office space, or raising funds from their customers (Ayer 2010). Because of all the various ways that corporations can support not-for-profits, this valuable stream of revenue can be essential to the success of any not-for-profit.

Conclusion

Regardless of the source of funding that a not-for-profit organization receives, some common challenges arise. In general, supporters of all kinds often like to support project funding, leaving organizations unable to support their infrastructure, sometimes losing autonomy, and drifting from their mission (Hall et al. 2003). No matter what trends we see in the future, we are likely to continue to have difficulties with long-term planning. We will constantly be searching for more funds and having to respond to a continually changing kaleidoscope of funding priorities from every conceivable kind of funder. In a world of constant funding flux, the consistent streams of revenue that come from true and successful partnerships can mean the difference between a groundbreaking not-for-profit and one that is constantly struggling not to lose ground. Although every not-for-profit struggles with fund-raising and planning how it will continue to fund itself, understanding basic statistics on streams of revenues can help organizations plan where they should be focusing resources and know how successful they are compared with their peers.

CHAPTER 6

Dimensions of Corporate Philanthropy and Partnerships

Because sport and recreation organizations receive less than 3 percent of donations from individuals (Hall et al. 2009) and more than 30 percent from corporate support (Easwaramoorthy et al. 2006), it is clear why organizations in the sport and recreation sphere value corporate partnerships. Sport and recreation not-for-profits receive a greater percentage of their revenue from corporations than any other type of not-for-profit does (Hall et al. 2005). Compared with other potential sources of funding, corporate partnerships tend to have excellent profit margins, especially compared with selling goods and services or providing membership benefits, which were discussed in the previous chapter. Therefore, a not-for-profit that successfully partners with a corporation can often invest in initiatives that may not be possible with any other type of support.

But only a small percentage of not-for-profits and corporations are truly able to call their work a successful partnership. For that reason, the partnership continuum introduced in chapter 1 is important. Most corporations spend most of their time, effort, and resources on philanthropy, a smaller percentage on sponsorships, and only a tiny percentage on partnerships. For a not-for-profit that is newly seeking corporate funding or that may not fit into the traditional mold of what a corporation wants to fund, some other areas of corporate philanthropy may be easier to obtain. In this chapter, we cover a few of the other major categories of corporate support, including corporate donations of cash, products, and services; corporate sponsorship; cause-related marketing; and employer-supported volunteering. Discussion of these methods highlights how corporations can leverage their stakeholders for support.

Corporate Support for Not-for-Profits

Corporate philanthropy and sponsorships are worth tens of billions of dollars in North America (Hall et al. 2005; Giving USA Foundation 2011). Despite the importance of corporate partnerships, a small minority of corporations and not-for-profits have arrived at true corporate partnerships. Corporate fundraising has become an essential source of funding for many not-for-profits, and a full 18.5 percent of charities in Canada now report soliciting funds from corporations (Ayer, Hall, and Vodarek 2009). In unpublished research on Canadian charities, I found that no type of fund-raising had increased as rapidly as corporate fund-raising over the last decade. For large organizations, corporate fund-raising has now become the single most popular type of fundraising; 55 percent of Canadian charities with more than $10 million in annual revenue report using corporate fund-raising (Ayer, Hall, and Vodarek 2009). Corporate fund-raising is a more popular fund-raising technique than personal solicitation, fund-raising events, or mail campaigns. For those involved with fund-raising, it is somewhat astonishing that for these large organizations, more fund-raisers ask corporations for money than ask their personal or organizational contacts for a donation.

Steven Ayer, President of Common Good Strategies, is coauthor of Chapter 6.

The outcome of this increased interest in corporate philanthropy is that more corporations report that their biggest challenge is the increasing demand for support (Muirhead 2006; Hall et al. 2009). To illustrate this conundrum, consider the Royal Bank of Canada (RBC), which in 2010 gave more than CDN$50 million to charities and gave an additional CDN$70 million in sponsorships (RBC 2011). RBC states that more than 80 percent of their giving is composed of grants of less than $10,000. Further, in 2010 RBC received more than 30,000 requests for funding (Melanson 2011). In the end, more than one-third of Canadian charities applied for funding from this one organization. The RBC Foundation was able to give grants to about 4,000 of those organizations, slightly more than 10 percent of those that applied. Many organizations of that size have only a dozen signature, or key, partnerships that they feature on their websites. For many organizations, figuring out how to become one of those key partners is the challenge.

This task is particularly challenging for small organizations that often have difficulty obtaining funds from corporations in the first place (Hall et al. 2005; Scott 2003; Easwaramoorthy et al. 2006). Attempting to reach the partnership level of the continuum could be discouraging to those organizations. Accordingly, to get the full value of corporate support, not-for-profits may want to start smaller on the donation side of the partnership continuum and build a relationship through smaller gifts before attempting to secure larger funds. Further, looking again at the RBC example, for many of the organizations that receive funds, $5,000 or $10,000 is a significant amount, especially if they can get similar amounts from multiple corporations.

Those unable to become signature partners should consider the other ways that corporations provide support. Many corporations provide essential products and services to not-for-profits at large discounts or free. Many corporations support employees who volunteer and donate in the community. An active donor or volunteer of your organization who works at a large corporation may be able to get additional funding for your organization just by submitting some basic paperwork to the corporation. Many corporations like to get their employees to volunteer with charities in teams. Creating an opportunity for employees of corporations to volunteer in a meaningful way may be a good way to receive more corporate support later.

How Do Corporations Give?

The Boston College Center for Corporate Citizenship conducted a survey of more than 700 businesses of all sizes in 2009 and found that 68 percent made cash donations or sponsorships, 60 percent made donations of in-kind goods and services, 57 percent supported employee volunteering, and 21 percent supported community investment. My colleagues and I (Hall et al. 2009; Ayer 2010) conducted a representative survey of 1,500 Canadian businesses and found that the majority donated cash (76 percent), many contributed goods (51 percent) or services (43 percent), many supported employee volunteering (43 percent), and a relatively small proportion raised money from employees

(18 percent) or used sponsorships (14 percent) or cause-related marketing initiatives. Large businesses of more than $25 million annual revenue were far more likely to use sponsorships or cause-related marketing initiatives. A small number also included support for not-for-profits in their supply chains, including raising money from customers or suppliers (22 percent) or purchasing goods or services directly from not-for-profits (14 percent). Because of the diversity of methods and types of giving, only a minority of large companies give solely through one department (Steger and Parsons 2006).

Another important question is how much a typical company gives. This difficult question may be best examined through metrics like giving as a percentage of profit or giving as a percentage of revenue. For example, in 2007 a study of many of the largest corporations in the United States found that the companies contributed 0.88 percent of their profit and 0.12 percent of their revenue (Coady 2007). The Conference Board surveyed 189 of the largest companies in the United States (Kao 2008) and reported a median contribution of 1.16 percent of profit and 0.08 percent of revenues. For public companies, finding revenue and profit numbers can be easy. For private companies, organizations like Dun and Bradstreet provide revenue estimates that can be used to determine an organization's capacity to give, which can then help determine the size of the ask that you should be seeking.

Why Do Corporations Give?

To understand the mechanisms that corporations use to support not-for-profit organizations, it is important to consider their motivations for giving. Often, different types of giving are used to support different motivations to different degrees. For example, although corporations may use donations to improve their reputations and, possibly, to increase sales, that goal is often secondary, whereas for cause-related marketing (in which a portion of each sale is donated to a cause or a charity) and sponsorships, that reputation enhancement can be the primary motivation.

Many researchers have examined the question of why corporations give. The major motivations that they identified are presented in table 6.1.

With all these various motivations for giving, note that large corporations indicated that only 7 percent of their donations were driven purely by commercial reasons (Coady 2009). On the other hand, 42 percent were classified as purely charitable, and 51 percent were identified as proactive community investment.

Of course, ultimately all these dimensions would be superseded by whether corporate philanthropy and partnerships drive profitability. Although answering that question is next to impossible, a few studies have shown that corporate philanthropy is associated with positive profitability. For example, a review of 167 studies that examined the link between corporate social responsibility and financial performance concluded that there was a small positive correlation between the two (Margolis, Anger Elfenbein, and Walsh 2007). Further, direct

TABLE 6.1   Major Reasons for Corporate Giving

Reason	Research source
It fits our company traditions and values or helps transmit our traditions and values.	Googins et al. 2009; Hall 2009
It improves our reputation or image.	Googins et al. 2009; Hall 2009
It's important to our customers or consumers or helps create loyalty.	CECP 2009; Googins et al. 2009; Hall 2009
It helps to recruit and retain employees.	CECP 2009; Googins et al. 2009; Hall 2009
It gives us a competitive advantage.	Googins et al. 2009
It helps us reduce business risks.	Googins et al. 2009
It allows us to get involved in the public policy debate.	Googins et al. 2009
It's part of our business strategy.	Googins et al. 2009
It helps manage regulatory pressure.	Googins et al. 2009
It's expected in our community.	CECP 2009; Googins et al. 2009; Hall 2009
It provides professional development opportunities for employees.	CECP 2009
It helps build government relationships and builds good-will.	CECP 2009
It builds media relationships that can aid a community should a public relations issue arise.	CECP 2009
It builds stronger, healthier communities, which are good for business.	CECP 2009; Hall 2009
It creates wealthier, more educated consumers who are more likely able to purchase the company's products.	CECP 2009
It encourages employee team building.	CECP 2009
The CEO or board has a personal interest.	Steger and Parsons 2006
It provides a license to operate.	Hall et al. 2009
It helps build new market knowledge.	Steger and Parsons 2006
It informs areas of innovation.	Steger and Parsons 2006
It builds acceptance of company presence when entering new markets or countries.	CECP 2009
It helps companies entering foreign markets brand themselves as part of that country's business community.	CECP 2009

contributions to charitable causes had the strongest linkage with financial performance of all dimensions of corporate social responsibility that they examined. An alternative though less rigorous way to examine the topic is to find whether companies themselves view their social responsibility practices as a driver of market differentiation. In that key measure, most businesses still have lots of work to do; fewer than one in four indicated that their corporate social responsibility (CSR) practices were successfully acting as a market differentiator (Googins et al. 2009).

Corporate Donations

As discussed in the previous chapter, in the United States corporate philanthropy is valued at US$15 billion per year (Giving USA Foundation 2011), and in Canada corporate philanthropy is valued at CDN$2.3 billion (Ayer 2011). In Canada, a large survey found that almost every large business made at least one donation to a not-for-profit (Hall et al. 2009) and that sport and recreation organizations were the third most popular kind of organization to support. Sport and recreation and promotion of general health and fitness are also popular philanthropic causes in the United States. Googins et al. (2009) found that health care, including nutrition and fitness, was supported by 33 percent of businesses' community investment programs and 48 percent of large businesses' community investment programs, lagging behind only education, which was supported by 49 percent of large businesses. Sport organizations were supported by 18 percent of community investment programs, and they were the only type of cause studied that was supported at a higher rate by small businesses versus large businesses. The margin was substantial; almost three times as many small businesses as large businesses reported supporting sport organizations.

As mentioned briefly in the previous chapter, estimates of the value of corporate donations are too low by a significant margin. In 2003 in Canada, corporations claimed $1.3 billion on their tax returns (Easwaramoorthy et al. 2006). In the same year, a survey of more than 10,000 of Canada's more than 160,000 charities and not-for-profits estimated the total value of corporate donations and sponsorships at $2.8 billion (Hall et al. 2005). Corporations were claiming less than half of their contributions on their tax returns. Although a portion of this total was likely sponsorships, most of the difference was not (Ayer 2011). This analysis, of course, does not reflect the many other types of value that corporations can bring, which are discussed in subsequent sections. No studies can accurately estimate the value of employee volunteering that is encouraged by the employer or accurately estimate the total value of goods and services donated or discounted to not-for-profits.

As our Executive Perspective with Scott Smith of Hockey Canada discusses, a not-for-profit needs to provide measurable value for a donation. If the organization does not do this, a partner will be unlikely to renew. For donations, which are not about marketing, not-for-profits can think of value as influence on the community as well. If you receive a large donation from an organization, you need to thank them appropriately and report to them about how you spent the money and any major goals that you were able to achieve because of their money. Corporations as well any other major funder will be unlikely to continue to support you if you do not account for using their money well.

Fund-Raising, Philanthropy, and Partnerships in Physical Activity and Health

Scott Smith
Chief Operating Officer, Hockey Canada

BIO

Scott joined Hockey Canada's head office in 1997 as the director of operations. He became the chief operating officer in 2007. As COO, Scott is responsible for the overall day-to-day operations of Hockey Canada, reporting directly to the president and chief executive officer, Bob Nicholson. Over the past 11 seasons Scott has led Hockey Canada in the hosting of national and international events such as the IIHG World Junior Hockey Championship and IIHG World Women's Hockey Championship, in the successful negotiation of a five-year broadcasting agreement with TSN/RDS, in the restructuring of Hockey Canada sponsorship opportunities and related activation and servicing, and in the advancement of the licensing and consumer products divisions. He sits on several boards and committees including the International Hockey Heritage Centre Board of Directors, the IIHG Marketing Committee, and the IIHG 100th Anniversary Committee.

MY VIEW ON PARTNERSHIPS

From Hockey Canada's perspective, partnerships between for-profit corporations and not-for-profit organizations like Hockey Canada are all about value. When we consider a partnership with a corporation, we ask what value we as an organization can provide to the partner corporation and, in turn, what value that corporation can provide back to us. It is easy to say, "OK, that company is going to invest $100,000 or $1,000,000," but our philosophy has always been that a good reciprocal exchange of value is the underlying key factor for a successful and sustainable partnership. By good reciprocal exchange of value, I mean one where the relationship is strong and will continue for a long time. If it is simply a donation without any measurable value, then you run into a two-phase risk over time of, first, becoming reliant on those funds (which will likely end) and, second, running the risk that the partner will not renew because the value to them is not worth the investment. So, we make sure that the value is sustainable within our mission, and we strive to deliver on what we promised.

In my experiences, I have seen organizations that compromise their own purpose and values in order to accept a contribution for financial gain but then spend the duration of the time in the relationship arguing and debating with the partner. It then ends and does not enhance the operation and programs of either organization.

PARTNERSHIPS AND RISK

I think there are situations where the corporation might not be of the same ilk or fit or share the message of the not-for-profit partner. In these cases, I'd suggest that these

(continued) ▶

(continued) ▶

are not the best partnerships. For example, in the 1990s when tobacco sponsorships were still allowed, we (Hockey Canada) had a policy that did not allow such sponsorships. Similarly, today, the International Ice Hockey Federation (IIHF) has a regulation that wine and spirits are not permissible for association. Hockey Canada has a similar policy. Even with beer—and we have a great partner in Molson—we are careful to make sure that that partnership is activated differently at youth and underage events.

To protect ourselves and make sure that our partnerships work, we have guidelines about how our brand can be associated with our partners. They are not overly stringent, but they do ensure that the presentation of our brand is in the manner that we want. A good example occurred at the 2002 Olympic Winter Games when one of our partners produced a number of our television and print advertisements that essentially made fun of or mimicked each of the other teams competing. It came to our attention that the other teams were using those messages as motivation for their teams to beat Canada. Thus, we then added to our guidelines that this use of our brand was not acceptable. So, we are sensitive and cautious about how and where our brand is presented. Another example would be our decisions to be cautious with partnerships with pharmaceutical organizations.

It is important to remember that there is a bit of a fiduciary responsibility for not-for-profit organizations to generate dollars to further their organizations and fulfill their mandate. If a potential corporate partner were to propose a substantial investment with your organization, it leads you to evaluate and consider such at a premium (even if there is some inherent risk with the association), where we would never compromise our brand. In general, I believe that managing the relationship side by executing and working with the partner to drive the partnership is the key philosophy. We like to think that we're Canada at its finest: humble but effective.

HOCKEY CANADA FOUNDATION

Philanthropy at Hockey Canada is largely run through our foundation, the Hockey Canada Foundation, through which we run events, engage our national team alumni, and involve key community people and partners to bring resources to help grow the sport, engage underprivileged Canadians, and build facilities for participation in sport. To date, the Hockey Canada Foundation has focused on events and alumni.

Currently, the foundation seeks to support six funds:

1. Canadian Hockey Foundation Legacy Fund
2. Canadian Hockey Foundation Heritage Fund
3. Canadian Hockey Foundation Flow-Through Fund
4. Canadian Hockey Foundation Operating Fund
5. Molson Olympic Hockey Fund
6. Named endowment funds

One of these funds has a corporate partner (Molson).

Most of the Hockey Canada corporate partners are invested in the Hockey Canada Foundation through their sponsorship investments whereby a proportion of their rights fees go directly to the foundation. We structured our partnerships this way to avoid situations in which a sponsor with a significant dollar investment is asked to sponsor a foundation golf tournament or gala for a much smaller amount or lose that event to a competitor who could then ambush the larger sponsorship. As such, we decided to assign a proportion of the sponsorship to the Hockey Canada Foundation. Of course, we never have enough for all our activities, but this works well to protect our brand and our top-level partners.

The foundation is under the jurisdiction of its own board of directors who administers the foundation (separate from the Hockey Canada Board). The foundation board is tasked with fund-raising for the various projects that the foundation supports, which is not an easy undertaking. Board members are selected based on two criteria. First, we want people who are associated with the game, have a passion for the game, and believe strongly in attracting young people to participate and play hockey for the betterment of their lives. Second, and also important, we seek members who have a strong background and network that is supportive of fund-raising.

A terrific example of how the foundation can really work is the recent partnership between the Hockey Canada Foundation, the Montreal Canadiens Hockey Club, and the City of Montreal to build rinks for youth, particularly underprivileged youth, in the city of Montreal. The partnership grew out of our 2009 gala held in Montreal. Our galas typically generate significant funds for the foundation. In 2009 we decided to invest a proportion of the funds raised to build an outdoor rink in the Verdun suburb of Montreal. The rink and programs to provide opportunities for underprivileged youth (e.g., Dreams Come True) was built, managed, and continues to operate with support from Hockey Canada, the Montreal Canadiens, and the City of Montreal.

ADVICE FOR MANAGERS IN NOT-FOR-PROFIT ORGANIZATIONS SEEKING CORPORATE PARTNERSHIPS

In general, I suggest a six-step approach:

1. Within your mandate, identify what you might be able to provide to a partner that would be of value to them. Think "assets."

2. Identify partners who you think might be able to help you achieve your objectives, who would be interested in the value that you can provide, and who could bring good intrinsic value to a potential partnership.

3. Initiate a conversation with them about how a partnership—not a donation— might work between the two. Emphasize value.

4. During the conversation, be very clear on expectations on both sides.

5. If you sign a partnership, deliver on the promises that you made.

6. If you sign a partnership, encourage your partner to keep the promises that they made.

(continued) ▶

(continued) ▶

GLOBAL APPLICATION QUESTIONS

1. What is reciprocal change in value, as Smith notes, in a partnership for (a) a for-profit partner and a (b) not-for-profit partner? Explain.
2. Smith emphasizes that public–private partnerships in sport are not risk free. From a risk management perspective, what would you recommend to any not-for-profit embarking on a partnership with a private-sector organization?
3. Discuss the importance of events in fund-raising for a not-for-profit.

Smith also makes the point that organizations have to be careful about becoming too dependent on one funder. A recent study of giving departments at large businesses (Steger and Parsons 2006) found that almost one-half were currently in the middle of a strategic review or just finishing one and two-thirds had significantly revised their programs within the last four years. Relying too heavily on one donor in an environment of such constant flux can have disastrous consequences.

One final point worth considering is that some corporations use corporate foundations as the vehicles of their philanthropic contributions to not-for-profits. In the previous chapter, we discussed that corporate foundations contributed US$4.7 billion to not-for-profits in 2010 (Lawrence and Mukai 2011). But among the 2,745 corporate foundations in the United States, just 12 of them, run by pharmaceutical companies to distribute donations of product, contribute $3.7 billion of that total. The remaining $1 billion is still a large amount, but nowhere as large as the original total. Canada has relatively few corporate foundations. In unpublished research on Canadian foundations, I was unable to identify more than 200 potential corporate foundations, and many of them would not grant to not-for-profits. Still, the RBC Foundation gives out more than CDN$50 million per year, so corporate foundations cannot be written off entirely.

In-Kind Donations of Goods and Services

Looking at donations of goods and services can be illuminating. Too often, not-for-profits think of donations of goods or services only as large products. But many financial institutions have free or much-reduced prices for financial transactions, particularly for not-for-profits. Professionals like lawyers or accountants may have discounted rates for not-for-profits that they would not offer to for-profit organizations. Many online web services offer large discounts to not-for-profits as well, whether it's a completely free basic package of a limited number of licenses like those offered by the software-as-a-service customer relationship management company Salesforce or a discount on survey software that could help not-for-profits do evaluations or identify the needs of its customers, supporters, or clients.

Similarly, many software companies choose to donate products to an organization like TechSoup, which distributes donated software to not-for-profits in the United States and Canada. TechSoup Global distributes tens of millions of dollars of software to organizations in more than 30 countries globally. Concerned Children's Advertisers, mentioned earlier in the book, noted the value of their partners' contributions to their success, including both the intellectual resources provided and the marketing assets, such as access to media, networks, and connections to other potential partners.

Many corporations choose to make in-kind contributions through an intermediary rather than directly to individual charities. Good360, formerly Gifts in Kind International, has distributed more than US$7 billion on behalf of hundreds of Fortune 500 companies since its inception. Good360 distributes hundreds of millions of dollars of goods per year, and it supported more than 120,000 community charities in the United States and around the world in 2007 (Gifts in Kind International 2008).

Some of the goods made available to not-for-profits are the following (Good360 2011):

- Clothing and footwear
- Toys and educational items like books and school supplies
- Building and home improvement supplies
- Health and beauty products
- Household items
- Software and technology
- Office products and productivity tools

In-kind donations are not always thought of as a robust area for partnerships, but instead as something that may be given as part of a strong partnership. But an interesting example from Good360 shows that this too can form the basis for a strong partnership. In 2007 Home Depot partnered with what was then called Gifts in Kind International to create the Framing Hope program, which diverts discontinued but otherwise usable goods from landfills to in-kind contributions for not-for-profits. More than 1,000 Home Depot stores are now involved. The program has donated US$80 million in products and 40,000 tons of goods to not-for-profits instead of sending them back to distribution centers or to landfills. More than 1,000 organizations have received products through this program.

Sponsorships

As was presented in detail in chapter 4, sponsorships are an important and growing element in marketing for corporations and in revenue generation for properties. Indeed, more than US$17 billion is spent annually in North America, and in excess of CDN$1.5 billion is spent on sponsorship in Canada.

Obviously, not every industry conducts not-for-profit sponsorships at the same rate. In my research I found that those most likely to be engaged in not-for-profit sponsorships were real estate and leasing companies, finance and insurance companies, retail trade companies, and manufacturing companies. Further, industry type also affected what form the sponsorship took. Manufacturing and retail trade companies offered sponsorships that included large donations of goods, whereas professional services and transportation and warehousing companies' sponsorships took the form of donation of services. Cash rich companies often make financial donations, especially if tied to a tax incentive.

In the United States, sport organizations are estimated to receive 68 percent of the total value of that contribution. In Canada, sport organizations received 50 percent in 2010 (CSLS 2011). In Canada, 57 percent of large businesses made a sponsorship investment in 2009 (Hall et al. 2009). In Canada, sport and recreation organizations were the third most popular type of organization to sponsor. Social services and health organizations, excluding hospitals, were the most popular type of organization to sponsor. For small businesses, sport and recreation organizations were the second most popular type of organization to sponsor, behind health organizations.

Cause-Related Marketing

Cause-related marketing is an appealing strategy for many companies that sell directly to consumers. The Canadian Tire Jumpstart Program discussed earlier in the book, created by Wilson Sporting Goods, the Boys and Girls Club, and ParticipACTION, involved creating branded basketballs, soccer balls, and footballs that were sold at Canadian Tire stores. The proceeds were donated to youth participation in sport and physical activity. The program is a good example of an interesting and effective cause-related marketing campaign.

Cause-related marketing does seem to be more effective for products consumed for enjoyment rather than products consumed for utilitarian purposes (Armstrong 2010). In other words, a cause-related marketing campaign would likely be more successful for a chocolate bar than for a box of staples. To build long-term relationships with customers, identify the specific amount given (Armstrong 2010).

The Boston College Center for Corporate Citizenship identifies five key principles of success for cause-related marketing (Boston College Center for Corporate Citizenship 2011):

1. "Treat cause branding like any other strategic business investment. Executives must take a purposeful approach to program development, maintenance and continuous improvement.

2. Support an issue, not just a charity. When a company focuses first on an issue and then brings in strategic partners, it is able to set its own course and mission.

3. Engage your employees' hearts and minds. Employees are the ambassadors of your program, and the emotion generated within your company is contagious, as it spreads to consumers.

4. Make your current assets work harder. Philanthropic dollars are limited, and to make them go farther it's necessary to consider a wide variety of other resources.

5. Earn the accolades. The line between informing and bragging is a fine one, and it varies by company and by audience. Let people know what you are doing. Be clear with your promotional and marketing efforts and about the amount of money going to a charity."

Employee Volunteering

Employee volunteering is an important additional potential form of partnership that not-for-profits should consider. Employee volunteering can seem like a relatively weak form of partnership, but conducted properly it can greatly enhance the relationship between two parties. For example, many corporations encourage their executives to participate on boards of charities. In more than one case I have seen this relationship result in large gifts from a corporation that had never supported the charity before.

Knowing that many of its employees volunteer and support a particular cause can increase the odds that a corporation will want to support a not-for-profit, even if the senior executives are not the ones who are volunteering. Remember that many corporations identified employee recruitment and retention as one of the key reasons for engaging in corporate citizenship behaviors.

In 2007 and 2008 my colleagues and I conducted a representative survey of Canadian businesses concerning their corporate citizenship behaviors (Hall et al. 2009). One of the areas that we identified was employee volunteering. Overall, 43 percent of the 1,500 corporations that we interviewed indicated that they supported employee volunteering. I outlined several major ways that corporations supported employee volunteers (the value in parentheses indicates the percentage of those that supported employee volunteering through the listed method):

- Allow employees to adjust schedules to volunteer (68 percent)
- Allow employees access to company facilities while volunteering (62 percent)
- Allow employees to take time off without pay to volunteer (51 percent)
- Provide financial donations to the organization that employees volunteer with (46 percent)

- Allow employees to take time off with pay to volunteer (43 percent)
- Have a company-sponsored volunteer event where employees volunteer for a cause selected by the company (26 percent)

Note that companies in the finance and insurance industries were most likely to support almost every type of employee volunteering measured. An example of an organization providing donations to those that their employees volunteer with is Bell Canada, discussed later in this book. The employee volunteer program is run by the True Sport Foundation, which helps Bell organize the donation of $500 on behalf of any Bell employee who volunteers at least 50 hours of her or his time to a local sport organization. This program has resulted in donations of more than CDN$700,000 annually.

Conclusion

This chapter identified a number of ways that corporations and not-for-profits can work together, and all of them can be valuable if used correctly. The not-for-profit must identify the resources that it needs, the valuable properties that it has, either because of their reach or because of their effectiveness at solving social problems, and the potential funders and partners who can help them reach their goals. No matter how strong a relationship is, remember the perspective offered by Scott Smith of Hockey Canada to avoid becoming overreliant on a partner and expecting that relationship to continue forever. Even when a partnership provides value to both sides, priorities for either partner can change. Finally, with all the competition out there for corporate support and effective partnerships, remember to focus efforts appropriately. Take the advice from this book and apply it effectively to ensure that your organization is one that breaks through and is able to achieve a successful long-term partnership.

CHAPTER 7

Role Models and Champions

An emerging consideration in the not-for-profit sport, physical activity, and health world is the concept of the role model, particularly with organizations whose efforts target youth in some aspect of their marketing and communications. These role models can be well-known celebrities (athletes, actors, singers, and so on) or they can be people whose notoriety may be less mainstream but whose efforts, personalities, and activities engage youth, or a segment of youth, in a meaningful way. These role models, by identifying with a specific cause, can become champions of particular causes or programs. On one hand, as a society we place great emphasis on building sport champions by developing world-class athletes, teams, and coaches. We are passionate about our favorite teams and professional athletes. We want to see them win tournaments and events, shave crucial time off their race performances, or perfect a victorious form. On the other hand, we need to consider championing sport (as a means of physical activity) and other ways to improve our society's physical fitness and health. Indeed, in most collaborative exercises, including partnerships, role models and champions, internal to each implicated stakeholder, are key elements to ensuring a successful collaboration (or partnership).

Celebrated professional and Olympic athletes can champion programs by increasing a partnership's local, national, and global recognition and support, and adding credibility and strength to the partnership. A good champion is connected to the partnership cause and able to communicate the partnership's messages effectively to participants and community networks. Athletes, executives, philanthropists, and others can use their skills to champion programs that have the broader goals of increasing health and sport participation.

Role Models

A prominent dictionary defines a role model as "someone worthy of imitation" and explains that "every child needs a role model" (Webster's Online Dictionary 2012). This definition is vitally important to this book and to those in health, sport participation, and physical activity organizations because it has no mention of size or reach. If celebrities such as singers Lady Gaga (34 million Twitter followers as of February 2013) and Justin Bieber (35 million followers) were the only role models, not-for-profit organizations would not be able to consider using role models. But the reality is that a terrific gymnastics coach whom 10 athletes may want to imitate is just as much of a role model. Good role models, from an organization's perspective, emulate the organization's goals and objectives and can help the organization or program by championing for recognition, funds, or greater participation.

Composition of a Role Model

Cruess, Cruess, and Steinert (2008) outline a number of key concepts, based on their research and previous literature, that are vital to any role model: (a) a role model has the ability to be a powerful teacher of knowledge, skills, and values; (b) a role model must be aware of the effect of his or her actions on others (positive or negative); (c) a role model must set aside time to facilitate dialogue with colleagues, reflect, and debrief with students; and (d) role models play an important role in our development as human beings.

Role models are not common, and really good ones are rare. In their research on teachers, Cote and Leclere (2000) noted that less than half of teachers at medical schools were identified by students as role models. We learn, they note, from observing role models and learning from them (Cote and Leclere 2000). But just because we believe a person to be a role model, she or he may not be an effective one. Researchers have noted a wide variance in performance of role models. Some encourage negative behaviors. Effective role models lead by positive example and encourage others to adopt positive behaviors and demonstrate integrity. Ineffective role models or those who affect negative behaviors and activities are the opposite and exude the opposite. Effective role models are able to adapt the results of their influence depending on the environment that they are in (e.g., speaking to a group of third-grade students versus a closed session with adults) to encourage positive outcomes and limit or eliminate negative ones (Cruess, Cruess, and Steinert 2008).

Role models are not mentors. Role models are not coaches. Role models are not managers. Mentors, coaches, and managers provide different services and are engaged in different relationships with their subordinates. A role model is an inspiring figure to his or her followers who leads by example (Cruess, Cruess, and Steinert 2008), whereas mentors, coaches, and managers are engaged in more interactive, tactical relationships. Role modeling occurs wherever and whenever the role model can be observed and followed. The role model could be the real person or an online or televised video version of him or her. Indeed, direct personal contact with the role model is not a necessary condition for the role model to be influential (Marx and Roman 2002), but the role model's record of success needs to be explicitly available if no direct contact is possible (Buunk, Peiro, and Griffioen 2007).

Role models, or those aspiring or on the track to become one, always seek both personal improvement and opportunities to demonstrate their competence, abilities, and values. These two efforts are well described in the case that follows. Other important tactics for role models include (a) realizing that they are in fact role models to others, (b) implementing time management strategies, (c) prioritizing those who follow them, (d) learning and communicating with colleagues and competitors, and (e) reflecting and learning from experiences.

The ability of a role model to improve performance in others and champion a particular vision is of utmost concern to organizations that might seek to develop, engage, or support a role model. As Marx, Ko, and Friedman (2009) report in their study, the effectiveness in supporting improved performance of a role model results from three drivers: (a) the role model must be perceived by followers as competent, (b) followers (or targeted people) must perceive the role model as a member of the social group or network (e.g., gender, race, culture), and (c) followers need to have high levels of awareness of the role

Partnership Highlight

A ROLE MODEL AND CHAMPION IN ACTION: ELIA SAIKALY AND FINDINGLIFE

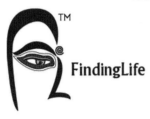

Reprinted, by permission, from FindingLife.

By any definition of role model that we have come across, Elia Saikaly is one. Elia created a movement (known as FindingLife) that has attracted and inspired many followers; his social media presence (as of February 2013) reports 2,281 likes of FindingLife's Facebook page, 3,174 Facebook friends for Elia, and 1,167 followers on Twitter. Elia's path to become a role model for thousands of youth began in spring 2005 with the death of Dr. Sean Egan, at the time a professor at the University of Ottawa, who died tragically during his summit attempt of Mount Everest. Elia was profoundly affected by Dr. Egan's death, even though Elia had only met Sean for the first time in Kathmandu, Nepal, in March 2005, three days before embarking on the expedition that would lead to Dr. Egan's death. Elia was Dr. Egan's camera operator on Everest, and they spent hours together each night interviewing in his tent. Dr. Egan became Elia's role model, someone whom he wanted to imitate and someone who inspired Elia's own desire to champion health, adventure, and passion in youth. As the leader of a 21-person, multinational research expedition, Dr. Egan wanted to use the platform of the world's highest mountain to spread his messages of physical fitness, health, and aging. Although his summit attempt had an unfortunate outcome, a number of positive benefits resulted from his effort, including his influence on Elia. Elia recalled during a trek to Aconcagua, "I think when Sean came along, and I actually got to know Sean . . . when I sat down with him at Kathmandu. I was so impressed. So moved. So motivated to change" (Saikaly 2009).

Following Dr. Egan's death, a large number of expedition members, including Elia, committed to carrying on his legacy, including a significant fund-raising effort known as Ad-Astra (the Nepalese version of one of Dr. Egan's favorite sayings, "Aim high") that raised money to build a school at a Nepalese orphanage in Dr. Egan's honor and a scholarship at the University of Ottawa in his name and managed by his family. But far beyond that was the effect on Elia, who changed his life drastically. He founded FindingLife and embarked on a new lifestyle and passion to affect others in a positive way.

FINDINGLIFE

FindingLife is a not-for-profit organization that combines adventure, education, technology, film, and charitable initiatives to inspire others to find their most meaningful life and spark positive world change. Through FindingLife, Elia has undertaken dozens of adventures over the past years to all corners of the globe, including his summits of Everest, Aconcagua, Kilimanjaro, Mount Kenya, Mount Elbrus, and many others. Elia and FindingLife have built relationships with schools, school boards, media partners, corporate partners, supplier partners, and key dignitaries to create a special organization that has become much more than a mountain organization as Elia had originally envisioned in 2009. Elia's first full-length documentary, *FindingLife*, is a spectacular piece that has been well received by Elia's target youth groups and has won numerous awards. FindingLife is not just an organization; it's a movement.

ACONCAGUA 2009

A trek up Aconcagua represented Elia's first effort to engage youth directly in a FindingLife adventure. Students in schools back in Ottawa followed the adventure through Skype and with integrated learning components in their curriculum. Students from one particular school who followed the expedition were surveyed before, immediately after, and one year following the expedition. Results showed that about 25 percent of the students involved had made positive changes in their lives a year later, linked to Elia, the team, and FindingLife.

MOUNT KENYA EXPEDITION 2011

Building from the success of Aconcagua and Elia's Everest expedition and successful summit in 2010, both of which had significant social media following, Elia had the vision to bring students with him on his next adventure. Partnerships were built with Garnier (title sponsor), Moving Mountains (charity partner in Africa), Adventure Alternatives (expedition management company), and the University of Ottawa (research partner) to create the 2011 Garnier FindingLife Expedition to Africa.

When the vision became a reality, the result was a three-week adventure with six Canadian high school students (selected by a competitive social-media-driven application process); six Kenyan high school students; two University of Ottawa students; and a team of media, researchers, filmmakers, and sponsors. A group of nearly 50 trekked up Mount Kenya, played a Kenya versus Canada soccer match, built two classrooms for a school in an impoverished area of Kenya known as Solio, and went on a safari. The effects, reach, and benefits of the adventure were significant at the levels of money and resources raised for charity, research completed, lives affected, and experiences gained.

> You know and we're coming up here and you're talking, we're talking about research and you're talking about role models, and you know so it's like, part of my brain shifts and has been working a lot on developing you know what I believe in, and who I am, you know what I think others can learn from all of this and you know I'm just afraid because I don't ever want to lose my passion. (Saikaly 2009)

GLOBAL APPLICATION QUESTIONS

1. Garnier is part of L'Oreal, a massive, successful, and global corporation. What benefit can they accrue by partnering with a small charity like FindingLife and a champion like Elia Saikaly?

2. What advice would you offer to Elia or not-for-profits of similar scope to FindingLife to attract private-sector partners?

3. Take some time to do a web search for Elia, FindingLife, and FindingLife Films. Report on what you find and note specifically any private-sector partnerships that have developed since this book was published.

model's success in domains where the role model's group is not expected to be successful.

Being a role model is not easy. It requires, as Elia demonstrates, passion, attention to detail, and a work ethic, particularly in the not-for-profit sport participation, health, and physical activity space. Elia has made enormous sacrifices but has achieved some wonderful things and partaken in some unique and truly life-changing experiences. The result would be similar for most role models and champions in the not-for-profit world of health, sport participation, and physical activity.

From Role Model to Champion

Role models can make good champions if they possess the necessary credibility, power, personality, willingness to commit resources, and passion for the related causes (Bryson, Crosby, and Stone 2006; Innes and Booher 1999). A good champion has some connection to your partnership and to the goals and objectives that you hope to accomplish, or to the community and participants that you hope to reach (Njaul, Mosha, and De Savigny 2009). With developed communication skills and established networks, good champions help promote your partnership message by attending events, reaching out to the media, and attracting a wider audience (Njaul, Mosha, and De Savigny 2009).

Does Your Partnership Need a Champion?

The success of a partnership can be determined by how well it is communicated to participants and supporters. Some authors (e.g., Bryson et al. 2008) suggest that champions are a necessary component of any partnership that hopes to be successful. In this regard, a program champion can increase a partnership's profile and build enthusiasm in the community and among participants. Bringing a champion on board in a collaboration or a partnership situation offers several key benefits.

Champions Bring Recognition

A champion can help communicate the partnership's goals and objectives and help the partnership gain recognition from participants, sponsors, and the media. This recognition can lead to benefits such as increased opportunity and ability to pursue sponsorship.

Champions Can Add Credibility and Strength to the Partnership

A well-known athlete or community leader who comes on board to champion a partnership is staking her or his reputation on a belief in the strength and success of the partnership. The Executive Perspective about Kevin Compton presented in the chapter is an example of this approach. The confidence in your partnership that champions demonstrate does not go unrecognized; participants and sponsors can associate the champion's achievements and values as representative of the credibility, strength, and value of the partnership (Njaul, Mosha, and De Savigny 2009).

Partnerships With the Public Sector and a Professional Sport Franchise: San Jose Sharks and the City of San Jose

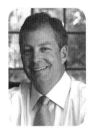

Kevin Compton

Managing Partner, Radar Partners, and Majority Owner,
Silicon Valley Sports and Entertainment

BIO

Kevin Compton is the cofounder of Radar Partners in Palo Alto, California. Radar Partners has invested in over 60 investment managers across asset classes such as real estate, timber, private equity, and distressed properties. These funds have performed well above their various benchmarks over the past decade. Kevin was a partner with Kleiner Perkins Caufield and Byers, one of Silicon Valley's most successful high-technology venture capital firms, for almost 20 years. Kevin and his partners invested in many of the most powerful and high-profile start-ups over the past 30 years, including Google, America Online, Compaq Computers, Lotus Development, Sun Microsystems, Intuit, VeriSign, Tandem Computers, Genentech, Citrix Systems, Netscape Communications, Amazon.com, and Juniper Networks. These companies employ over 300,000 people, have annual sales in excess of $100 billion, and carry a public market value of more than $300 billion. Kevin has been featured in many technology publications, has been profiled in *Fortune*, *Forbes*, and *Inc. Magazine*, and has been ranked as one of the top venture capitalists in the world over the last decade. The *Forbes* "Midas Touch" ranking of top investors has named Kevin as one of the top private investors in the world on numerous occasions and has ranked him in the top 10 three times. Outside work, Kevin enjoys spending time with his family, playing hockey, and working in youth sport. His passion for sport extends into the professional area as well. Kevin is a co-owner of the National Hockey League San Jose Sharks, the American Hockey League Worcester Sharks, and Silicon Valley Sports & Entertainment.

MY VIEW ON PRIVATE SECTOR NOT-FOR-PROFIT PARTNERSHIPS

I am a business guy and I take that approach to all aspects. A partnership is about making a deal that both sides win on. That is the key. It is really quite simple.

Specific to partnerships that support causes such as health, youth, and similar good things, I think that anyone who pushes back against companies or organizations who are funding these things should be completely ignored. That drives me crazy. Companies are trying to do a good thing, investing money that they do not need toward a cause to help make the world a better place. Just take the example of McDonald's. I think all the work that they did in supporting the Olympics and kids over the last 20 years has effectively changed their menu in a positive way.

(continued) ▶

(continued) ▶

Maybe I'm a free-market goofball, but let me reemphasize my point on the support of the business world for causes. The support of corporations opens eyes to a problem or an issue. It provides support for those organizations. The last thing, in my view, anyone would want to do is to shut that off.

SILICON VALLEY SPORTS & ENTERTAINMENT PARTNERSHIP WITH THE CITY OF SAN JOSE

My team, Silicon Valley Sports & Entertainment, runs a number of properties including the San Jose Sharks, the HP Pavilion, and Sharks Ice (skating facility). In the case of the HP Pavilion (a 17,600-seat arena that is home to the Sharks, concerts, and other events), the city owns the building, and we have a 100 percent operating relationship with them through HP Pavilion Management, our arena management company.

We've approached the city many times over the 18 years we've been in the building. We have a strong relationship. Each side keeps a reserve fund, to which each contributes quarterly, and both sides must agree in order to use the reserve fund. As landlord, they likely have the stronger voice, but we've never really had a situation where one side has wanted to do something that the other has not wanted.

Updating the scoreboard a few years ago was a very large expenditure. We both put in millions. As a business guy, the timing and process with the city is always a challenge. But my guys are very good at getting things done and working efficiently to make the partnership work. For example, our lease comes up in 2015, and we're already 80 percent done with the renewal (June 2011). It is a closed market because we're the only anchor tenant, so we're in a good position. We don't have to stay but probably will.

The partnership has worked very well over the past few years and I think there are two keys to this:

1. Being way ahead of the issues. We work together to make sure we identify in advance the issues that we'll face.

2. Having the mutual advanced capital fund that both parties have control over. As I noted, both the city and our group pays into it every quarter, and neither can use any of those resources independently. This prevents misuse, and it is always clear how the resources are used. I believe that both sides put in the same amount.

I know that the city is pleased with the relationship as well. I had a chat with the mayor recently in which he stated that other cities are asking about the program and the partnership and wondering how and why it works so well. The mayor also informed me that the two buildings that we manage for the city, HP and Sharks Ice, are the only two city facilities that are cash-flow positive.

ADVICE FOR MANAGERS IN NOT-FOR-PROFIT ORGANIZATIONS SEEKING CORPORATE PARTNERSHIPS

A couple of things are vitally important for me here:

1. Business people are interested in working with organizations that measure outcomes and results. They prefer measurement and outcomes to groups who

come in with a proposal and offer that just says, "We are trying to help," "We are doing a good thing," or "We are a good cause." So, my advice is to make sure that you walk in with a business case. Have clear outcomes and measurements. For example, we coached 1,000 kids, we've seen parents report changes in their kids X percent of the time, we have seen a decrease in city violence, and so on.

2. Stemming from the previous point, show documented positive outcomes in people's lives. Stress how these outcomes will help the company by providing a better pool of employees in their community in the future. Make sure that your outcome measures are true and that you can show credible positive results.

GLOBAL APPLICATION QUESTIONS

1. Compton is an owner of a pro sport team. Why, in general, would a pro sport team be interested in public–private partnerships?

2. Compton has a strong view on the importance of the business world working with causes. Although some disagree with him, many people agree. Why would someone support his view?

3. Compton describes how his team prepares well in advance in its dealings with the city. This is an example of understanding the public-sector partner. What other things should a private-sector organization be prepared for in working with a public-sector partner?

Champions Generate Greater Community Awareness and Support

A good champion is often tied to networks of like-minded groups and individuals who can contribute to spreading the message in the community. By increasing visibility of the partnership in new networks, the champion can reach new contributors for additional funding or resources. For example, Women's International Boxing Federation's Intercontinental Junior Lightweight champion Esther Phiri takes on the role of championing empowerment and participation of women and girls in sport through her work with sport-for-development organizations and her sponsorship agreements in Zambia (Meier and Saavedra 2009). Esther Phiri is recognized in her community, and females throughout the country have embraced her championing efforts.

The National Hockey League's San Jose Sharks have benefited from the championing work of Kevin Compton in building their external partnerships (see Kevin Compton's Executive Perspective in this chapter). In the case of Compton, his reputation as an elite financier and businessman in Silicon Valley provides the Sharks with the champion they need in dealings with the City of San Jose and other partners. Compton and all champions increase public recognition and credibility of the organization's work and grant better access to new cultural or regional groups that may be beyond the organization's regular demographic. As an individual, Compton has the personality and passion for his team. As a successful businessman and member of the local corporate community, he has the resources (financial, human, and network) needed to drive his organization's partnerships. Finally, as principal owner of the team, he has the credibility and power to drive these partnerships internally and externally. But Compton is just one type of effective champion. Champions are of many styles and types. Indeed, a good champion is often a vocal and visible face of a partnership. A champion can be an individual (an athlete, celebrity, philanthropist, or business executive) or an organization that works to support and promote a cause or program.

Athletes as Champions

Individual athletes can be involved in partnerships to help build and enhance programs and give back to communities. Even the casual recreational athlete may become an intermediary because charities are increasingly using sport as fund-raising events (Wood, Snelgrove, and Danylchuk 2010). Because high-performance sport events and athletes have the ability to draw huge audiences (e.g., one billion people watched Brazil and Germany live in the 2002 World Cup final), tying athletes to partnership programs can have enormous influence (Right To Play 2008a).

Some athletes are active in establishing partnerships through the creation of their own foundations by using their own visions, goals, and missions. For example, the Mike Weir Foundation's partnerships benefit disadvantaged children, and the Steve Nash Foundation promotes health and wellness in underprivileged children and development efforts in Africa. Celebrity athletes such as Ronaldinho, David Beckham, and Michael Jordan, as Right To Play (2008a) pointed out, can have popularity that "transcends cultural and political borders," allowing them to use their celebrity status to reach worldwide audiences.

In 2006 Chelsea soccer striker Ivorian Didier Drogba and Marseille's Nigerian player, Wilson Oruma, were part of an Africa-wide Roll Back Malaria Partnership between the Global Fund to Fight AIDS, Tuberculosis, and Malaria and Sumitomo Chemical (a mosquito-net manufacturer) (Right To Play 2008a). Drogba, Oruma, and 10 other high-profile athletes used their soccer celebrity status in a television campaign delivered in French, English, and several African languages to educate viewers across Africa about the risks of malaria and the use and benefits of mosquito nets. The TV clips combined soccer action clips with education messages and included an eight-second space at the end of the clip to add a local malaria campaign message (Right To Play 2008a).

A note of caveat: Athletes can be effective champions who can raise a partnership's profile, but professional athletes are also role models, especially for children. In selecting a professional or celebrity athlete to champion your program, you should consider the athlete's lifestyle and habits. A partnership addressing cancer may not want to select an athlete who smokes cigarettes, and an obesity partnership may want to avoid someone who has an appetite for fast food and soda. A good champion should live in a way that is consistent with your partnership's messages.

Partnering to Reach
Multicultural Markers

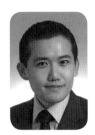

Camon Mak

Former Director, Newcomer and Multicultural Markets,
Royal Bank of Canada

BIO

With over 12 years of experience within the financial services sector, my current assignment is to lead RBC's Multicultural Markets portfolio within the Canadian Banking division. In this capacity, I work with various groups to ensure that the bank's products, services, and overall value propositions are compelling to newcomers.

MY VIEW ON SPONSORSHIPS: USING PARTNERSHIPS TO IMPROVE RBC'S RELATIONS WITH MULTICULTURAL POPULATIONS

RBC has long recognized the importance of the growing client base made up of new Canadians. RBC reflects Canada as a whole with our interest in attracting newcomers. Historically, our client base was concentrated from North America and Europe, but we see significant changes in newcomer arrivals from China, India, Philippines, and beyond. Since 2000 RBC has been promoting a strategy that goes beyond banking to consider what we at RBC can do for newcomers in Canada. Through our strategies, we demonstrate how RBC understands new Canadians. We've reached out to help newcomers find gainful employment and make good connections in Canada. For example, to reach out to the largest newcomer group, from India, we form partnerships to connect with the local community through activities and sports that are familiar from back home. At RBC the connections with the local community reflect our desire to show that we understand new Canadians' needs and wants. Developing greater brand affinity is one consideration, but in that effort we also want to make an impact in local communities by helping the kids of new Canadians connect and bond through RBC's supported opportunities. In essence, partnerships help us connect the RBC brand to the community.

PARTNERSHIPS IN ACTION: RBC'S SUPPORT OF CRICKET IN CANADA

As part of RBC's commitment to amateur sport in Canada, we work with the cricket world to help develop talent and provide participation opportunities in one of Canada's fastest growing sports. Our work with partners to develop cricket opportunities is part of a deliberate attempt to reach out to newcomers through a sport they are familiar with and to give kids ways to connect to their community. RBC's Wicket Cricket program provides free cricket equipment to local schools (equipment was delivered to

(continued) ▶

(continued) ▶

over 1,100 schools, and more than $250,000 in grants were made to municipalities, recreation centers, and cricket clubs to support the growth of cricket in Canada). RBC's in-school programs are aimed at increasing schoolchildren's awareness of cricket in schools in Ontario and British Columbia. We want to bring cricket alive for students and parents by hosting cricket day camps, funding cricket facilities, and providing other cricket-related opportunities.

RBC's commitment to amateur sport and desire to connect with local communities is also exhibited in our hockey partnerships. Through our Play Hockey program, we drive greater brand awareness through specific media pitches. For newcomers, the program aims to increase understanding and affinity of the sport. We recognize hockey as one of the key pillars of Canada and a way to help newcomers adapt and integrate in Canada. Again, this initiative is about connecting our brand to the community.

Both the cricket and hockey partnerships are part of how we help newcomers connect to us, connect to Canada, and connect to Canadians. We see the potential in helping integration happen through grassroots sport participation. We also spread the message that sports are not just for established Canadians, but that new Canadians can participate and enjoy community sports too.

We've been extremely satisfied with the way that our sport partnerships in cricket and hockey have played out. When you consider our partnerships, the return on investment, public relations value, and mentions from press have far surpassed our expectations. We think our partners (the schools, local associations, municipalities, Ontario Cricket, and Cricket Canada) are also happy with our partnerships; they are getting free equipment, more spotlight, higher participation rates, and greater sponsorship awareness.

CHAMPIONS IN ACTION

RBC has been aggressive in bringing in cricket superstars (including Sunil Joshi and Wasim Akram) to help promote cricket and reach out to newcomers. When we brought in cricket champions to promote the RBC Wicket Cricket program, we saw an increased presence of newcomers in our local branches. We've also seen that our program helps parents connect to their kids by passing on their own love for cricket. We are investing in a sport that new Canadians are familiar with, and we see the benefits. One surprising element was that, with the partner champions on board, our strategy is reaching more than just South Asian newcomers; the champions are helping us connect to broader multicultural groups as well as established Canadians.

By bringing in the cricket stars, it became clear that they are pillars of the community. We realized that you can rarely find a better way to connect with the community; Sunil Joshi and Wasim Akram brought the spotlight to our partnerships and showcased our brand affinity in new Canadians' home countries (as media picked up stories about our initiative that were delivered in India, Pakistan, and beyond). Champions help drive better engagement and increased awareness of our amateur-level programs and partnerships.

PARTNERSHIP LESSONS: RESPECTING THE BOTTOM LINE

From a business perspective, for RBC to engage in a partnership or to sponsor or support a new initiative, we need to consider what the opportunity can bring to RBC. Our RBC Foundation does support philanthropic and social causes (e.g., $100,000 funding to increase access to cricket facilities), but RBC's corporate side needs to consider the return on investment before we consider new partnerships. Too often, we are approached by not-for-profit groups that have not considered how RBC could benefit from being part of their initiatives. The lesson for public and not-for-profit groups is that in connecting with a private organization or requesting a sponsorship, the "ask" should identify benefits for the private organization to become involved. With the increasing scrutiny from shareholders and other corporate gatekeepers, not-for-profits must try to think of the private business perspective in terms of how the opportunity relates to the private partner's return on investment: How will the partnership drive more business? How does it help develop greater brand affinity? Without clear answers about how the partnership can benefit the private partner, even programs that get off the ground might eventually be cut or abandoned. The profit mode takes precedence, and the partnership must therefore drive down to the bottom line, especially in times of recession. Partnerships need to be results driven. The appropriate question is not "How does the request benefit the not-for-profit or public group?" but "How does the partnership help the private business bottom line?" A good partnership needs to bring value to the private partner by helping it to meet its ultimate objectives.

GLOBAL APPLICATION QUESTIONS

1. Mak is Director, Newcomer and Multicultural Markets, at RBC. Why would a bank have such a position and department?
2. Mak notes that partnerships are a way to help build a brand, RBC's brand. How does this work?
3. In your view, why has RBC decided to partner with cricket not-for-profit organizations?

Gatekeepers as Champions

Champions can bring partnership programs into new regions and to different demographics that are unfamiliar to you and your partners. Good champions may also possess linguistic skills and cultural knowledge that helps them be embraced by certain regional and cultural groups. By using a regional or cultural insider as a champion, the partnership is better able to access and communicate with the populations that it hopes to serve. For example, to reach out to newcomers from China, India, Philippines, and beyond, the Royal Bank of Canada (RBC) recruited cricket superstars (including Sunil Joshi and Wasim Akram) as champions for its Wicket Cricket program. They highlighted RBC's partnership and better engaged newcomers with the RBC brand.

A Good Champion Is Connected to the Partnership Cause

The champion with authentic ties or a vested interest in the partnership's goals or objectives is seen as more credible. With professional and Olympic athletes as champions, the love of sport and the commitment to a healthy lifestyle is often enough of a connection to drive their willingness to get involved in a partnership (e.g., more than 350 athlete ambassadors support Right To Play programs without compensation). Turning to health champions, as a cancer survivor, actor Cynthia Nixon is a good champion ambassador for the cancer charity Susan G. Komen for the Cure.

A Good Champion Is Tied to the Community or Participants

Local leaders, celebrities, professional athletes, and role models in smaller communities often step up to the role of champion, showing their commitment and personal ties to the community where a partnership is delivered. For example, National Hockey League player Andrew Brunette champions the Teddy Dore Memorial Fund, named in honor of his late friend who succumbed to cancer in 2008. Brunette created a local hockey equipment bank for underprivileged kids in his hometown of Valley East, Ontario, Canada. With the support of the NHLPA Goals & Dreams fund, National Hockey League Players' Association members like Brunette are able to give back to their communities and contribute to grassroots hockey programs.

A Good Champion Is a Proficient Communicator and Networker

Champions can bring recognition, but good champions are also often recognizable community leaders, large-business owners, philanthropists, local heroes, or celebrities. With top-notch communication skills, a good champion is able to reach out to participants, media, and other groups who may be interested in the missions and objectives of your partnership. Good champions are also normally linked into networks that can offer additional support, promotion, and resources. For example, as a champion for the Maasai Wilderness Conservation Trust (MWCT), a partnership between young Maasai leaders and professional conservationists, actor Edward Norton promotes the partnership through his marathon participation. He communicates his efforts and raises MWCT's profile through blogging and other forms of social media in running and development networks, aiming to get more people involved by recruiting MWCT team runners who can further spread the message and raise more funds for the partnership.

A Good Champion Shows Up

A good champion is a visible face of the partnership. Often busy in their own professions, champions have the difficult task of committing time to be spokespeople for the partnership and to be present at races, tournaments, events, and galas. The champion also has to be available to speak for television, radio, web, and newspaper media. A good champion has to show up ready to "live" the partnership in the way that they communicate and in the way that their choices reflect a healthy and fit lifestyle.

How Do You Recruit and Retain a Champion?

Just as each organization's goals, values, and missions are considered when establishing a partnership, the individual champion's goals and purpose for participating in the partnership should be clearly communicated. Champions normally have a natural stake in the partnership, but organizations are reminded to give back to the champion while being respectful of the champion's boundaries (e.g., time and priorities). The champion's strengths and commitment should be recognized formally when possible through appropriate internal and external communication. The champion should be part of the partnership communication plan, which should include an exit strategy and plan for succession if the need arises.

Champions in Action

In physical activity and sport, champions can promote messages of wellness and healthy behavioral changes, and they can draw new participants to sport programs. Many partnerships have been successful in building champions for their programs. Two organizations, ParticipACTION and Right To Play, are successful examples of incorporating champions in their efforts.

ParticipACTION

Established in 1971 with a mission to be "the national voice of physical activity and sport participation in Canada," ParticipACTION is a leader in getting Canadians more physically active (ParticipACTION 2010). The development of *The Partnership Protocol* (as presented in chapter 2) demonstrated ParticipACTION's desire to lead and champion public–private partnerships as a way to fight the obesity epidemic and support increased physical activity in Canadians. As O'Reilly and Foster (2010) described, "ParticipACTION not only had adopted partnerships with the private sector effectively in its own activities but . . . also sought to champion the broad use of these partnerships in sports and physical activities, first in Canada and then throughout the world" (p. 2). With strong leadership under Kelly Murumets, ParticipACTION acted in a championing role, calling on support from public (e.g., Sport Canada and the Public Health Agency of Canada) and private partners (e.g., Kellogg and Coca-Cola) to reduce levels of inactivity and support health and fitness pursuits for all Canadians.

Right To Play

The sport for development organization, Right To Play, is a choice example in embracing champions in their programs. The goal of the Right To Play Champions program is "to improve the lives of children in some of the most disadvantaged areas of the world using the power of sport and play for development, health, and peace" (Right To Play 2009). With personal donations and a commitment to support Right To Play's initiatives and mission, the champions are key fund-raisers made up of business owners, executives, and

Championing Partnerships:
Promoting Life-Skills
in Aboriginal Youth (PLAY) Program

Julia Porter

Deputy Director, Education and Aboriginal Initiatives,
Right To Play Canada

RIGHT TO PLAY

Reprinted, by permission,
from Right To Play.

BIO

Right To Play is a humanitarian organization that uses sport and play programs to improve health and develop life skills for children and communities in 23 countries around the world. In June 2010 Right To Play, with generous funding from the Ontario Ministry of Aboriginal Affairs and other charitable donors, initiated the Promoting Life-Skills in Aboriginal Youth (PLAY) program in partnership with Moose Cree First Nation and Sandy Lake First Nation. The objective of the PLAY program is to build on the strengths of Aboriginal youth and their communities, while supporting the value of culture and identity. Since June 2010 Right To Play has partnered with 38 First Nations and one tribal council across Ontario to implement the PLAY program.

The PLAY program, a multifaceted program tailored to the specific needs of each community, is designed in partnership with the community and aims to support children and youth to develop and strengthen essential life skills. Before implementation, community members participate in a thorough needs assessment that guides the design of the program.

MY VIEW ON PARTNERSHIPS

Partnerships are a critical component of any development work, whether it is done locally or internationally. To carry out any sort of program, organizations need to form partnerships and collaborate. Three integral types of partners are the key to success in the PLAY program:

1. First Nation partners: The PLAY program exists only because First Nation communities request to partner with Right To Play to implement it. Having a strong and well-established partnership with each First Nation is essential in ensuring that the program is locally driven and meets the needs of the community.

2. Funding partners: We reach out to partner corporations, individuals, philanthropic foundations, and government ministries to secure essential funding for the program as well as to generate local and international awareness and enthusiasm for the program.

3. Implementing partners: We work with a large variety of organizations, communities, and institutions in an effort to create the most effective programs. We try to select partners with visions that are aligned and with skill sets and ideas that will add to creating a unique program.

Partnerships are essential to success. But it is important for organizations to be selective when developing partnerships to ensure that all parties are aligned in working toward a common goal and have a clear understanding of their role in the partnership. Without this, the partnership and the program can fall apart.

The Ministry of Aboriginal Affairs (MAA) approached Right To Play (RTP) with the concept of applying the experiential education model that Right To Play uses to remote First Nation communities in northern Ontario. RTP advertised this new program at regional health conferences and, with the assistance of the MAA, opened an application process. A significant number of applications were received. RTP together with the MAA decided which communities would benefit most from the program. The two selected pilot communities were Sandy Lake First Nation and Moose Cree First Nation. Since 2010, interest in the PLAY program has significantly increased among First Nations, so a formal committee has been established to review applications and select partners. The PLAY program is currently implemented in partnership with 38 First Nations and one tribal council across Ontario.

When working with First Nation communities our experience has taught us that establishing trust and building a relationship with the community is imperative. As with designing a program overseas, the needs of each partnering First Nation must be the top priority when designing the program. This means ensuring that the program is both sensitive to and inclusive of local cultural practices, activities, and beliefs. RTP works side by side with the chief and council. Each partner works to select local community mentors to manage and direct the program and local youth staff to support the children involved in the program. The chief and council also commit to paying 50 percent of the salary of the community mentors as well as a portion of the youth staff salaries. Moreover, RTP has enlisted the support of a number of local partners (elementary schools, high schools, child protection services, community health services, and so on) who contribute to the implementation of the program by offering in-kind contributions of venues, equipment, food donations, staff support, and training.

RTP offers remote ongoing supervision, support, and assessment of the program from Thunder Bay and Toronto, as well as in-person supervision and support every two months during a staff visit and training. But the day-to-day operation of the programs is left in the hands of locally hired staff, who have the responsibility and the opportunity to create, modify, tailor, and implement the program in the way they see as most appropriate.

FORMULA FOR SUCCESS

The programs that have resulted from the partnerships between First Nations and RTP have been met with overwhelming support from all involved. This initial success can be credited to the work that the local community mentors, chiefs, councils, the RTP

(continued) ▶

(continued) ▶

staff, the MAA, and the University of Ottawa (Human Kinetics Department) did in preparing and designing the PLAY program. All levels of the community, from children and youth through to teachers, parents, and members of the band, were involved in thorough needs assessments conducted by RTP staff and U of O professors. The first objective was to take time to build strong relationships in the community and better understand their priorities in terms of programming. This approach allowed RTP to tailor the various components of the program to each community based on their need. After completing the needs assessment, Right To Play staff and U of O staff returned to each community to share their findings, to ensure that their understanding was correct, and to confirm that their action plans were deemed appropriate. Next, each community began a recruitment and hiring process for youth to staff each program.

BUILDING CHAMPIONS AND ROLE MODELS

To run the After-School and Summer Sun (day-camp) programs (two of the core components of the PLAY program in each community), RTP needs approximately 6 to 20 youth and 3 to 8 elders from each community. All youth who are hired participate in an interview process before selection and then participate in a three- to five-day intensive skills-building workshop. One of the intended outcomes of the PLAY program is an increase in confidence and life skills among youth. Employing youth, training them, supervising them, giving them an opportunity to take on a leadership role, and offering ongoing one-on-one and group feedback all contribute toward this outcome. RTP aims to have the youth enhance their skill sets and become positive role models in the community. Additionally, RTP is striving to incorporate elders into the activities by having them work directly with the children and share their life experiences and information about the culture. RTP hopes that by training youth to work with the children and enlisting the support of elders in the implementation of the program, children will be surrounded by positive role models who encourage and support them, model positive behaviors, and create an environment that helps children and youth believe that positive change is not only possible but achievable.

OVERCOMING CHALLENGES AND LOOKING FORWARD

At the start of the program, many members of the initial First Nation partner communities voiced hesitation. Community members questioned the value of the program or the commitment of the organization. They spoke of a long history of visiting NGOs and organizations from the "south" who arrived with solutions in hand but never took the time to get to know the people or the issues. They spoke of many organizations and individuals who had come with promises and quickly left without fulfilling them. Overcoming these historical concerns takes time, and RTP is constantly working to demonstrate our commitment to listen, collaborate, build relationships, and stay the course.

Despite the positive feedback to date, RTP would like to see more active parental involvement, both in the program and with their children. RTP is still struggling to find ways to engage parents in every community. The most successful community programs are accompanied by the highest levels of parental engagement, and this is what RTP is striving for. The programs are continually improving, but overall the feedback received to date has been much better than predicted.

ADVICE ON PARTNERING WITH FIRST NATION COMMUNITIES

We have learned a few key lessons that we try to live by when working in partnership with First Nations. New lessons are added each week, but the following five seem to be consistent:

1. Be aware of how little you know: No matter how much time you have spent in a particular First Nation, it is essential that you remain grounded and remind yourself of how little you truly know. Each First Nation is unique and has its own history, culture, and beliefs. Don't apply lessons from one First Nation to another. Instead, enter each community with an honest understanding of how little you know. Be humble and genuinely seek to learn about the intricacies of the community you are working with.

2. Invest real time and energy in being in the community: It is important to invest a lot of time and energy in really getting to know the community, the culture, and the chief and council. You should not plan to implement a program immediately; instead focus on developing strong relationships and spending time in the community. Be sincere, show interest, and demonstrate your commitment to each community.

3. Never stop seeking guidance and support: Look to the community for guidance and to other local community leaders and organizations who have been there before you. Right To Play is new to partnering with Aboriginal communities and has a lot to learn. We look to other examples of successful individuals, organizations, and institutions and seek constantly to learn and grow from the experiences of others.

4. Collaborate: Collaborate as much as possible by bringing as many motivated minds together as you can, all working toward a common goal.

5. Hire locally: There are many creative minds in the community; build from their strength, experience, and understanding and be prepared to learn and be inspired in the process.

GLOBAL APPLICATION QUESTIONS

1. Right To Play partners with MasterCard and Roots, two private-sector corporations. Why would each (respond separately) be interested in partnering with Right To Play?

2. Porter outlines funding and implementing partners. What are the differences between the two?

3. What does Porter advise when partnering with not-for-profit organizations in First Nation communities?

philanthropists from a wide range of backgrounds in investment, commerce, law, sport, health, media, communication, and other areas. Athlete ambassadors can also support the champions. Through partners in the National Hockey League Players' Association (NHLPA) and alumni associations, Right To Play programs have welcomed current athletes (e.g., Andrew Ference of the Boston Bruins) and hockey legends (e.g., Darryl Sittler, Wendel Clark, and Jim McKenny), among other media and management-level supporters. In partnership with the Ministry of Aboriginal Affairs (MAA), Right To Play's partnerships with First Nation communities in northern Ontario recruit and train youth to act as champions for after-school and summer day-camp programs. The youth, with the support of community elders, work, champion healthy behavior, and become positive role models for community youth.

Conclusion

Recruiting a champion, or better using a role model, can help deliver part of your partnership's marketing and communication strategy. By increasing recognition, credibility, and strength, the champion can generate greater community awareness and support. With proficient communication and networking skills, champions may be viable ways to reach out to regionally, culturally, and linguistically diverse participants. Good champions need to be authentically connected to the partnership cause and have some ties to the community or participants. Athletes can be effective champions if they are willing to get involved, driven by the love of their sport or community. Organizations like ParticipACTION and Right To Play, among others, have been effectively using champions in meeting their goals and objectives in sport, physical activity, and health. Other organizations may encourage their executive and leadership teams to champion programs that are part of their philanthropic and corporate social responsibility.

CHAPTER 8

Leveraging Corporate Social Responsibility to Partner With Corporations

Corporate social responsibility (CSR) is a relatively new concept in business management that refers to a private-sector organization, typically a corporation, that invests resources, effort, and time into improving its local city, province or state, country, and planet. Just as its name infers, CSR is about organizations' taking interest in their society and taking ownership of their environment. Originally, CSR was a new and different approach to corporate involvement in society, but today most organizations have some part of their budgets and activities devoted formally and annually to CSR initiatives and related endeavors. The topic is therefore relevant to partnerships and this book. Indeed, CSR has particular importance to marketers working in the not-for-profit health, sport participation, and physical activity sectors because it provides these organizations with another tool to use in attempting to build strong partnerships with private-sector organizations as part of larger strategies to increase their organization's resource base.

Given the highly tactical nature of this chapter, it is organized as a mixture of expert perspectives and specific tactical recommendations directed toward managers and marketers in not-for-profit health, sport participation, and physical activity organizations.

Introducing CSR

In brief, CSR is the philosophy that corporations can and should give back. It (see Love 2006) can be described as contributing to the communities in which an organization functions, which is good for business because "as the health of the community system improves, so does the performance of the firm within the system" (p. 61). In their work about FINA's World Aquatics Championships, Seguin, Parent, and O'Reilly (2010) outlined a strong benefit, through CSR, for sponsors of megaevents. Specifically, citizens of the host city responded positively to organizations who were sponsors of the megaevent in their city. The same set of benefits, we argue, is certainly possible for not-for-profit organizations in health, sport participation, and physical activity.

CSR has been effective for many corporations in improving business, reputation, and brands because it (a) demonstrates to that corporation's communities that the company is locally involved and linked in to their host communities; (b) provides tangible or perceived value to members of those communities who, in turn, link this back to the corporation through purchase behaviors, positive word-of-mouth, or changes in perceptions; and (c) has the ability to communicate that the company manages itself in a socially responsible and environmentally friendly way (Holland, 2003).

A few specific quotes from the CSR literature will help explain its role in organizations further, particularly with respect to partnerships. First, Robins (2005, p. 99) notes that private-sector companies respond to society's demand to "accept costs and responsibilities which may well be remote from their commercial focus and from which there may not be any identifiable return in revenue." Thus, although it may not directly affect their business or be directly part of their function, an expectation has been created that private-sector companies of a certain size should be involved in CSR-related activities. Second, Carroll (1999) proposes that corporations taking a CSR approach should "strive to make a profit, obey the law, be ethical, and be a good corporate citizen" (p. 290). This view, as written, places considerable responsibility on any corporation and its management. These two factors further emphasize the opportunity for not-for-profit organizations to leverage CSR in building partnerships with the private sector. Third, in their seminal work on CSR, Varadarajan and Menon (1988) outline in detail that CSR benefits for the corporation are long term in nature and related to reputation, branding, and the marketing concept (i.e., changes that will result in returns in terms of sales in the long term). Their work signals that both sides should be prepared to make significant investments over long periods to allow CSR to provide the economic, noneconomic, or mixed benefits that are possible (Drumwright 1996), including the ability of CSR to have a positive influence on the views that consumers have of a corporation and their intent to purchase that corporation's products or services (Mohr and Webb 2005).

Corporate Perspective on Partnerships

At noted, CSR is a concept, construct, and strategy developed by corporations for corporations. As such, not-for-profit management needs to understand this perspective and embed it in any private partnership efforts that they undertake. Dave Moran, vice president for Coca-Cola and responsible for such partnerships in Canada, provides his views on this topic in the following Executive Perspective.

Integrate CSR to Attract Partners

As observed by Dave Moran in his perspective, not-for-profit organizations seeking to partner with for-profit entities need to understand the for-profit partner and provide partnership opportunities that can help the private-sector partner achieve their objectives. In the case of high-profile not-for-profit organizations, corporations often seek partnerships and provide all the activation resources required to produce a successful partnership. But these situations with high-profile not-for-profit organizations (e.g., International Olympic Committee, World Health Organization, American Medical Association, and so forth) are rare. The reality is that most not-for-profit organizations have to work extremely hard to find, maintain, and renew partnerships with the private sector. Certainly, most not-for-profit organizations have fewer partnerships than they would like. Thus, to help these not-for-profit organizations find additional private-sector partners, we provide four examples of adoptable tactics. There are certainly other approaches and adaptations of these four, but our hope is that they will provide direction, ideas, and models to follow.

Role of Corporations in Partnerships: Leveraging Corporate Social Responsibility

Dave Moran
Director of Sustainability and Community Investment,
Coca-Cola Canada

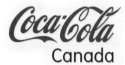

BIO

Dave Moran is director of sustainability and community investment for Coca-Cola Canada. One of Dave's responsibilities is creating long-term partnerships to further the company's sustainability goals. One example of these partnerships is a multiyear million-dollar partnership with the World Wildlife Fund to protect and preserve key watersheds in Canada. Before joining Coca-Cola, Dave worked as a senior political advisor.

PARTNERSHIPS AS A SOURCE OF OPPORTUNITY

For me, partnerships between the sectors represent a tremendous opportunity for us, as a society, to solve real problems with real solutions. When you think about conquering major global issues like obesity, water shortages, and climate change, we all need to work together to overcome these challenges. And, when I say together, I am referring to engaging governments, nongovernmental organizations, the private sector, and other stakeholders. If you consider the "big three" stakeholder groups, we at Coke view them as the golden triangle when it comes to working together on these issues. In simple terms, the "big three" graphic refers to the importance of the interaction of the three most important sectors of organizations to generate the ability to make larger contributions to our society (see figure 8.1). Indeed, if we want to tackle major issues like world hunger or terrorism, all three sectors must be involved and contribute.

As figure 8.1 depicts, these three groups need to work together or at least support each other and not hinder the other groups if we are going to make significant progress on these major issues. Clearly, governments and NGOs have vital roles but so does the private sector, which provides resources and, more important, reaches into communities to enable access to people everywhere.

Now, additional stakeholders will affect this relationship. For example, I like to say that all of our partnerships and programs related to causes like active living or water need to be "critic acceptable," that is, we want to do things in a way that will allow them, for the most part, to be acceptable to those groups who hold alternative views. Highly linked to being critic acceptable is doing things that the public would support. Other stakeholders that are vital to us include our customers and our shareholders.

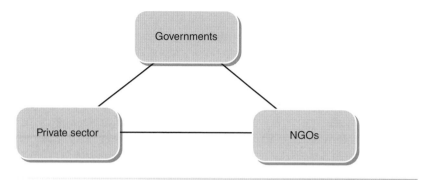

FIGURE 8.1　The "big three" stakeholder groups.

NORTH AMERICA

Specific to the area of change in active living, physical activity, sport participation, and health, there is not a consensus in North America amongst the three groups in the golden triangle. In my view, the role of the corporate sector is more established in the United States than it is in Canada, but for both countries that consensus is still missing. Let me explain by presenting what I see to be the view from each of the stakeholder groups.

Governments: The main challenge here is that for the most part they are not willing to work with the private sector. This, coupled with the fact that they do not have enough resources to fund all the projects and programs related to key issues, means that they cannot do everything. So, instead of partnering with the private sector, governments typically go the route of regulation, where rules are put in place. From a resource perspective this works because regulations have no direct costs attached. But, from an effectiveness perspective, they do not. For example, how do you regulate a 15-year-old kid off a couch or away from a screen? In these health-related areas, regulation has a role to play, but programs, activities, and promotions need to accompany it.

Nongovernmental organizations (NGOs): Many NGOs believe that governments should solve all problems and that their funding should come only from those sources. This view may be biased, but in many cases it is true. And, it doesn't work, because governments do not have enough resources to invest and, in fact, they have less and less that go to NGOs as core government funding goes up for health and education. So, many have been pushed to look to other sources, including sponsorship. Everyone in the NGO world first looks to those perfect sponsors, like Mountain Equipment Co-op (MEC), but they are tapped out quickly and do not have the budgets to support many things. So, perfect sponsors are limited in volume and often small. This has two impacts: financial and reach. You need the big sponsors to aid in global problems and have to deal with the fact they are not perfect. Consider the banks financing the tar sands projects or food and beverage companies supporting health programs. But they do provide the resources and access to people everywhere.

Sponsors: I like to take the view of Michael Porter (Harvard professor) here. The era of philanthropy is dead. Corporations want to be socially responsible. But it needs

(continued) ▶

(continued) ▶

to have a link to the overall business plan of the organization. If not, it tends to be short term or fail. Specifically, companies are seeking to make a difference in areas that affect them, where they can view their support as a real investment with societal and corporate benefit, and where their consumers would expect them to be. To do that, the investment has to be tied to the business plan, where real engagement results from real investment. In our case at Coca-Cola, we only offer beverages, so all of our products include water, and because the transportation costs of water are so high, the vast majority of our products are made locally around the world. So, it makes business and societal sense for us to get involved in projects and work toward the long-term sustainability of water and watersheds. Investing in water projects makes sense for society, for us as a corporation, for our partners, for our customers.

SELECTING PARTNERSHIPS

It is important to understand the process that corporations go through when deciding what partnerships to get involved with. It is quite simple, really. It is about business strategy. For us, we look at partnerships that affect core areas in which we operate: water, lifestyle, hydration. We also look at health-related issues because health affects consumption of our products. Active living is one of these areas.

Generally, businesses also need to prioritize, in my view, partnerships with the public sector and NGOs. We need to convince them of the value of these partnerships, demonstrate the resources we bring, and outline how we can do so in a constructive win–win manner. We need to demonstrate that we, the corporate sector, have a positive role to play. Specific to sensitive areas like active living and health, we have to do so in a careful manner, but there is a role for us to play and a positive one. There are many great examples of this already, including our partnership with ParticipACTION.

THE FUTURE OF PARTNERSHIPS

A key thing for me is to start—and this is happening in pockets—to increase the dialogue between governments, NGOs, and businesses. We need to talk, plan, and work together to come up with common solutions to major problems. At the very least, we have to get out of each other's way and allow things to happen. So, we need much more serious discussions. We need certain NGOs to open up to the private sector. We need the public to be more supportive and aware of how partnerships can be done in a responsible way. We need to address the problems and not symptoms of the problems.

In the case of Coca-Cola, we're doing our long-term 2020 planning right now. Many corporations are. It is an ideal time to develop partnerships that have long-term objectives related to major social issues and integrate them into our business plans for the next decade. Active living is there. Sustainable watershed is there. Others could be. Partnerships could be expanded. Corporations can be socially responsible and still profitable but it takes planning, collaboration, and effort.

Specific to partnerships related to active living, the future for me is engaging youth, getting them off screens, and doing active things. I could see a government supported, private-sector-funded, NGO-run program with major impact.

GLOBAL APPLICATION QUESTIONS

1. Coca-Cola is a global player in partnerships with the not-for-profit sector, including the International Olympic Committee and FIFA. Do you think that this is a good business strategy for the organization?

2. Moran outlines what the private sector brings to partnerships with the not-for-profit sector. What does he say? Do you agree?

3. Moran says, "The era of philanthropy is dead. Corporations want to be socially responsible," supporting Porter. What is the key point that he is making?

Recognize Your Cause

In chapter 2, as part of *The Partnership Protocol*, the disconnect (the gap between the private-sector partner's image and that of the not-for-profit partner) concept was introduced. It is important to consider that the greater the disconnect, the greater the potential value is for the private-sector partner and, in turn, the greater the cost (or premium) should be for the private sector to enter into the partnership. This point is important to all partnerships. Before seeking corporate partnerships, a not-for-profit organization needs to understand its cause and the value proposition that it offers to potential partners. For example, if your cause is associated with health and youth, you have a potentially strong proposition for corporate partners in food and beverage, biotechnology, pharmaceuticals, and other industries seeking those associations. In these cases, if the not-for-profit organization decides to take the risks inherent in such a partnership, the private-sector partner needs to invest at a level appropriate to the risks taken and the value being provided back.

This point supports the recommendation that any not-for-profit organization should research, benchmark, and internally investigate their organization, their equity, their competition, and their environment to understand clearly what their cause is (e.g., childhood obesity, smoking, safe sex) and what associations, images, and attributes they possess (e.g., access to youth, healthy image, charity). In terms of specific steps, a multilayered research approach is required, including review of internal strategic documents and surveys and interviews of the public, stakeholders, volunteers, and employees.

Build Your Own Properties

The second suggested tactic, and one that has been growing considerably in use in recent years, is the idea of a developing or partnering with a third party (e.g., agency, event management firm) to develop your own property that links strongly to your cause and attributes and that, more important, provides your corporate partner with a platform to activate and achieve their objectives.

Note that the key element that distinguishes an owned property from other properties is that the organization who seeks the benefit also is the owner or creator of that property.

A quick observation of promotions and events reveals that many such properties are in existence. Good examples can be found in Canada where corporations create such owned properties to link to the sport of ice hockey, Canada's most popular sport, and speed skating, Canada's most successful Olympic sport. For instance, Canadian Tire, a large retailer, has built its marketing association around hockey with a number of efforts including Canadian Tire Hockey School, a program that provides opportunities for youth to learn the game from NHL stars. A second example is Intact Insurance, who has worked with its partner Speed Skating Canada to create a property known as Day on Skates, a daylong activation held in a variety of Canadian cities whose goal is to engage Intact's brokers (Intact is a large insurance company) and encourage locals to try skating and be more Canadian.

In general, owned properties can be very successful but are also inherently risky because corporations must invest considerable time, human resources, and financial resources to research, create, and implement the owned event. This process may take months and, in some cases, years. Although the event may be successful, failure would cost the corporation both time and resources. Thus, to date, many owned properties are created by third-party agencies engaged by large corporations who can afford to risk the financial resources upfront and who have the background and experience in event management to manage these properties successfully.

Organizations may also create their own events to attract sponsors. An example is the Heritage Classic, an outdoor hockey game played at a larger outdoor baseball or football venue each January. The organization, the National Hockey League in this case, has created the property with an aim to attract corporate partners. Although less plausible for most small not-for-profit organizations in health, sport participation, and physical activity, they do exist (e.g., ParticipACTION's Sports Day in Canada) and can be very successful.

Leverage Role Models

Chapter 7 provided a case study and the conceptual background on champions and role models in health, sport participation, and physical activity. The chapter included the case study on Elia Saikaly, FindingLife, and Garnier. As was demonstrated, champions and role models are valuable tactics by which a not-for-profit organization can engage its target markets amongst much competition. Thus, the tactic here is simple: Identify a series of potential role models, evaluate their ability to help the organization outperform its competition, and select one (or more) to engage in the marketing communications efforts of the partnership.

Bring Other Partners to the Table

When a CSR initiative is undertaken by two partners, an opportunity may be available to engage additional partners in the effort. As noted, most (if not all) organizations seek some sort of CSR activity to benefit their reputation in the communities in which they exist. Thus, an existing partnership with active and reputable partners could provide an opportunity to partner with an additional corporation. Indeed, interest would likely be significant. Similar to a partner who takes on the role of a cosponsor, a second or third sponsor who joins has reduced risk (i.e., the property already has a strong title sponsor) and the ability to partner with the other sponsor as well as the sponsee or property.

How CSR Can Improve Partnerships

The previous section discussed adopting CSR or related tactics to attract corporations to partner with a not-for-profit organization. This section focuses on partnerships that are already in place and how CSR can play a role in making the partnerships stronger and more likely to continue into the future.

Image Transfer for Your Corporate Partner

As introduced in chapter 4, an important element in successful corporate sponsorship is developing and activating sponsorships that allow for the transfer of images from the not-for-profit partner through the sponsorship association to the corporate partner (i.e., consumers alter their views of the image attributes of the corporate sponsor to be more aligned with the associations that the not-for-profit partner brings to that partnership). This process is well established in the marketing literature (see chapter 4), and thereby a relatively straightforward three-step approach is recommended here for the managers of the not-for-profit partner.

Step 1 is to work with your corporate partner to identify which attributes of your organization (the not-for-profit partner) are of interest to the private-sector partner. Particular effort to include the CSR elements of the contribution of the corporate partner will be included. This step could involve a review of previous decisions, results of consumer studies, and interviews with key decision makers at the corporate partner. Step 2 involves reviewing the activation, media and communications plan, and tactical elements of the sponsorship to focus resources on achieving the transfer of the images identified in step 1. Finally, in step 3, a control process is developed to track and evaluate the effectiveness of the partnership in achieving the identified image transfer elements (with requisite benchmarks, metrics, and methods). The results of these evaluations are shared with the corporate partners and changes are made, where needed, to improve the effectiveness of the partnership. Lauren MacDonald provides some context on Gatorade's view on partnerships in this regard.

Being True to Your Organization and Its Priorities

Lauren K. MacDonald

Marketing Manager, Gatorade at PepsiCo Canada

BIO

Lauren is a graduate of Queen's University, School of Business and holds a bachelor's of commerce (honors) degree. During her studies, she spent a year abroad in Germany. She also completed three internships in Germany, where she gained marketing training at BMW and L'Oreal.

Lauren joined PepsiCo Canada straight from Queen's and began her marketing career on the Quaker Oatmeal cereal portfolio. Her next assignment was on the beverage side of the business where she worked on the innovation team launching new products. After two years with the Canadian business, Lauren made her first international move to the UK where she joined the PepsiCo's snack division and became brand manager of Walkers snacks. Lauren spent three years in the UK in various roles within the snack division and then made another international move to the Middle East, where she became senior marketing and sales manager for the Dubai royal family's real estate organization, where she managed iconic brands like the World Islands and the Palm Islands. In the two years following, Lauren returned to where she began her career and accepted the role of Gatorade marketing manager with PepsiCo Canada.

KNOWING YOUR PRIORITIES AND TARGETS

Gatorade's number one priority is to support athletes, ranging from grassroots to professional levels. Being clear on that priority makes it easier to evaluate the numerous requests (I receive more than five calls per day) for products or other forms of donation or sponsorship. With the limited Canadian budget, Gatorade needs to stick to its main objective and consider opportunities only when there is direct benefit in growing the number of athletes who experience their product.

Gatorade maintains partnerships with all professional sport leagues, has developed several grassroots partnerships (e.g., with Hockey Canada), and provides product samples and education about products directly to target athletes. Partnerships with endurance races are considered important opportunities to trial new products (e.g., G-Series Prime) to athletes before and after the races. With our G-series products, our bull's-eye target is the 15-year-old male competitive athlete, and we have an overall focus on performance athletes. PepsiCo has a policy not to market to children under 12 years old.

Most of our agreements are in the form of three-year, locked-in, sponsorship-type deals in partnerships that meet our goals and objectives in a real way. We want to reach our target athletes, so we are selective in choosing our partnerships. We look for specific exposure opportunities rather than take part in a maximum number of events. We normally require exclusivity (to be the only sport drink supplier) and can add other type of promotional requirements such as a presence on websites or banners.

Currently, our partnership list is a mile long. Each partner must fit with Gatorade's objectives, and the partnerships must make sense as a way to reach the 15-year-old male athlete at a "point of sweat." By understanding your organization's objectives and where other organizations are coming from, you can build mutually beneficial relationships.

GLOBAL APPLICATION QUESTIONS

1. MacDonald notes that Gatorade often provides product to its not-for-profit partners. Why is this the case? Why would certain for-profit organizations prefer to offer product rather than cash investments?

2. PepsiCo has a policy not to market to kids under age 12. Why would PepsiCo have such a policy?

3. MacDonald noted that Gatorade's partnership list is "a mile long." Is that list too long?

Return on Investment for Your Corporate Partner

This tactic is intuitive and almost not worthy of dedicating space to it. But because the corporate partner needs to achieve a positive return on investment (ROI), we believe that it is worth including. The suggested tactic is simple: Adopt a framework of ROI for the corporate partner in all aspects of the management of the partnership and its CSR elements. Any decision, activity, or action that the not-for-profit undertakes in relation to the partnership (e.g., activation, evaluation, meeting with partner, and so forth) must be done with this approach clearly in mind. That is, at every level and at every step, the not-for-profit organization should focus on providing a return for their partner on the investment that they make in the partnership and the not-for-profit. A simple example would be media efforts related to the partnership. In this area, the not-for-profit would seek to include a quotation from a senior executive of the corporate partner in every newspaper article about the partnership. The focus of this return, whether brand, sales, or other, needs to be determined before the process begins.

We also suggest that the management of the not-for-profit partner put in place efforts to enhance the nonfinancial (e.g., volunteers, in-kind contributions of products or services, word-of-mouth effort) resources supporting a partnership that are based on its CSR benefits and strengths. An example of three such tactics is included in table 8.1.

TABLE 8.1   Specific Tactics to Attract Nonfinancial Resources for Activation

Tactic	Details
Role model recruitment	Recruiting well-placed people as role models, representatives, or board members on or related to the partnership
Value in-kind sponsors	Pursuing in-kind sponsors for needed nonfinancial resources such as media time, products (e.g., bottled water for a charity run), and services
Social media	Developing a social media platform that allows proponents of the associated cause to pass on their views in a more influential way

Examples of CSR in Partnerships

To provide further learning and evidence about partnerships involving CSR, brief backgrounds of a few examples are included here.

Canadian Breast Cancer Foundation CIBC Run for the Cure

The CIBC Run for the Cure is an annual event held in Canada that developed from a partnership between CIBC (Canadian Imperial Bank of Commerce) as the corporate or private-sector partner and the Canadian Breast Cancer Foundation as the not-for-profit partner. The event website (www.runforthecure.com) noted that the CIBC Run for the Cure, first held in 1992, raised more than CDN$30 million in 2011 and was held in 59 communities in 2012. The website describes the CIBC Run for the Cure as the largest single-day volunteer-led fundraising event in Canada dedicated to raising funds for breast cancer research, education, and awareness programs. The event is a grassroots-focused activation in which families and friends of those who either have died from or have survived breast cancer seek pledges for the annual run. All benefits go to the Canadian Breast Cancer Foundation, which invests the funds in research and programming.

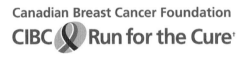

Reprinted, by permission, from CIBC Run for the Cure.

Scotiabank AIDS Walk for Life

Scotiabank, another large Canadian financial institution, provides us with another example of a CSR-based partnership with a not-for-profit organization. In this case, three not-for-profit partners work with Scotiabank, the corporate partner, to raise money for AIDS research and programming.

The not-for-profit partners include the Canadian AIDS Society, ACT (AIDS Committee of Toronto), and the Positive Living Society of British Columbia. The walk first took place in 1986, and it became the Scotiabank AIDS Walk for Life in 2008. Besides Scotiabank, a number of other corporate partners participate (see www.aidswalkforlife.ca for details).

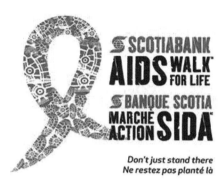

Reprinted, by permission, from ScotiaBank AIDS Walk for Life.

Shoppers Drug Mart Weekend to End Women's Cancers

A major pharmacy and drugstore, Shoppers Drug Mart, has partnered with (see www.endcancer.ca) the Princess Margaret Hospital Foundation (the charity arm of a large Toronto hospital), the Alberta Cancer Foundation, and Jewish General Hospital in Montreal. The event, held in Toronto, Alberta, and Montreal involves

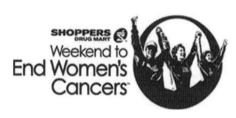

Reprinted, by permission, from Shoppers Drug Mart.

teams of individuals raising dollars and doing a variety of walks (of various distances) over the weekend. More than CDN$45 million has been raised for cancer research since 2005.

How to Leverage
Corporate Social Responsibility

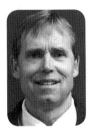

Paul Melia

President and CEO, CCES, and Chair of the Board, True Sport

BIO

Paul Melia has been a key leader at the Canadian Centre for Ethics in Sports in its work on values-driven sport for more than 15 years. He has an extensive background and expertise in the development and implementation of public awareness, education, and social change campaigns for a variety of health and social issues. Paul is currently the president and chair of the True Sport Foundation, a national charitable organization that promotes values-driven sport. He is also the cochair of the True Sport Secretariat, the central coordinating office for Canada's True Sport Strategy.

MY VIEW ON PARTNERSHIPS

I think that a partnership between a not-for-profit organization or cause and a for-profit corporation is good when it can be a win–win for both partners. The only thing that we at the Canadian Centre for Ethics in Sport (CCES) are concerned about is how the for-profit company is using the partnership to alter their image and affect ours. We, as not-for-profits, need to guard against undesirable results. For example, in our business of antidoping, supplements are a huge issue. They are the source of some banned substances that cause many athletes to have positive doping tests. If we were to get involved in a partnership with a supplements manufacturer, we would be appearing to endorse that supplement company. They would launch marketing efforts, and we would be viewed as supporting the company and the supplements. Given that our position is that if athletes are going to use supplements, at the end of the day they need to know what they are putting in their bodies, we need to be super careful and consider the risk to our integrity. Our top asset as an organization is our integrity, and if we traded on that, the risk would be huge for us. So, we don't. Every not-for-profit organization has that value or a similar one at the core of what they are about. When they have partnership with a corporation, they have to be careful. So, I think about examples of partnerships with riskier partners like Coke and Pepsi and the backlash that sometimes arrives. Some organizations have managed that relationship well and have kept the negative link out of it. An example is the SOGO Active program with Coke and ParticipACTION. But even then, at times it spilled over, and the connection was there. But again, I think we can't be so wrapped up in our own principles that we prevent ourselves from getting in relationships that allow us to do our work and fund our programs. When you think about those types of partners, tobacco is clearly offside. But others are not and can be considered. In our case, we won't partner with tobacco, alcohol, pharmaceuticals, and gun companies. This is where I am very big on the ethical decision-making process and looking at it from all the stakeholders' perspectives and how they are likely to react and see the relationships. I try to use that as a test to assess whether to go forward with a partnership or not.

A NATIONAL VIEW ON PARTNERSHIPS WITH THE PRIVATE SECTOR

When we look at—and I think this is true from a company perspective as well—partnerships from a national level, we are interested in nationally based partners but partners who are in the local communities as well, like a Tim Hortons or a bank. So, for us, to be able to have a partnership with a company that has retail outlets or offices in many local communities is a great basis for a relationship. For example, we're (CCES and True Sport) in discussions with Canada Post (Canada's postal service) right now, and in my view they would be a perfect partner because they exist in every community. They are still a gathering place. People interact there, and we can use that network to get our message out to influence change because they have the channels that we don't.

When looking for national partners, one of the first places that we find common ground is the values that we have (integrity, ethics, fair play). And organizations are interested in those values. We're talking to a major bank right now, and they want to reach out to Canadians through all mediums to connect with Canadians in all corners of the country around what it means to be Canada and what the values are that make us Canada. The very value that True Sport stands for is what they want to get across and use to inspire a social change in our sport system.

TRUE SPORT AND PARTNERSHIPS

A charitable foundation started by CCES, True Sport is by our definition

> a social movement powered by people who believe that sport can transform lives and communities—if we do it right. True Sport members across Canada are committed to community sport that's healthy, fair, inclusive, and fun. True Sport members stand together against cheating, bullying, aggressive parental behaviour, and win-at-all-costs thinking.

To date True Sport has largely been funded by the Canadian Sport Awards, which it manages on an annual basis with financial support from the government of Canada.

True Sport has some corporate partners on the corporate social responsibility side. Bell Canada and the McConnell Foundation were both originally on board as community partners and had a goal to address barriers to access for youth to hockey and soccer. Each made an annual contribution in excess of $1 million. Bell also asked us (and still do) at True Sport to run their volunteer employee program. That program was structured so that for any Bell employee who volunteers at least 50 hours to their local sport organization, Bell would donate $500 to that organization in the name of the volunteer. The program has been very successful, and Bell contributes about $700,000 annually. Investors Group has just signed on for a similar program at $200,000 annually.

(continued) ▶

(continued) ▶

In the case of Bell and Investors Group, True Sport is the partner, not CCES, because we can provide a tax receipt, and both corporations viewed True Sport as a better fit in terms of values, alignment, and risk.

Our work with McConnell still goes today on the Community Development Fund with such things as paying for registration to sport program for kids who cannot afford it. But we found that this approach was not sustainable, so we tried to find a way to remove barriers to access in a sustainable way. Our belief is that we need to reduce these barriers in the long term to achieve True Sport's objectives. This led us to the Community Foundations of Canada. In this interesting organization, each member community has a foundation that reaches out to wealthy Canadians in that community and builds an endowed fund to support projects to build stronger, more resilient communities. We've said that one of the best ways to do this is to build a healthy, vibrant sport system in these communities to address crime, vandalism, health problems, and so on. To prove this, we're currently carrying out four pilot projects across Canada in hopes that we can demonstrate that this approach, through a foundation, is effective, demonstrating that you can have great results on the issues that you address with a well-designed program, that in turn will enable us to attract partners.

SHARE VALUE—AN IMPORTANT CONSIDERATION FOR PARTNERSHIPS

I have recently done some reading on this concept, and I now view this as the next stage from corporate social responsibility (CSR). CSR comes from a place in a company's mind where they say, "We're in competition with other companies in our category for consumers, so one way to distinguish ourselves is to associate with a cause that we think our consumers support or would like to see supported. So, if we align with the cause, it will, in theory, endear us to our consumers and they will choose our product over the competition's products." We looked at this to find how we could ensure a win–win for a company and the cause. I think implicit in a win–win is that the association will cause no harm to either partner.

From my understanding of share capital, it includes a notion that the company is building a relationship with the cause or issue in the community to build an ecosystem where what they do to give back produces a better quality of life or addresses basic conditions that allows their consumer group to become stronger. The company can generate more value from their product if it can directly affect their bottom line as opposed to developing differentiation from the competition.

We at True Sport have been playing around with the idea of share value. Because we're based on a number of values and principles, one idea is to give back to the community through the pursuit of inclusion and access to sport for all. On the partnership level, we've had some preliminary discussions with Giant Tiger, whose primary market is blue-collar and value-shopping Canadians. So we're currently asking ourselves whether we can build a relationship with Giant Tiger that will contribute to True Sport in such a way that kids and families become customers of Giant Tiger.

CHAMPIONS IN PARTNERSHIPS

Champions can be extremely helpful if you get the right champion. They have to be iconic Canadians who embrace, reflect, and display the values that True Sport is all about. Therein lies the risk because a champion who violates the values can do a lot of damage to your brand and image.

We talk about champions in our work because we see the power of high-profile sport people in Canada. Think about Clara Hughes, Steve Nash, Wayne Gretzky, and others like them—people who live those values and personify the very things that we are, if we can get them involved. Their ability to connect people to a message helps a partnership immensely. They are much more effective as champions than a CEO or administrator is.

ADVICE FOR MANAGERS IN NOT-FOR-PROFIT ORGANIZATIONS SEEKING CORPORATE PARTNERSHIPS

I have two key things to suggest:

1. Understand the business objectives of the corporate partner. If you can understand their objectives and business model, you can look at whether your not-for-profit can contribute to those objectives. In the example of Giant Tiger and True Sport, we've been looking at the idea of doing things in the community aimed at engaging community members to drive traffic to Giant Tiger stores through a coupon, a financial incentive, so that it is addressing the business needs of the company, providing benefits to the community (i.e., goods at a reduced price), and providing some value for sport (e.g., equipment exchange, getting families out to participate).

2. You have to be conscious of and place appropriative limits on the relationship so that your brand and your organization are not used in other ways by the corporate partner. Establish those limits upfront and in writing so that both partners are protected and aware.

GLOBAL APPLICATION QUESTIONS

1. Melia, a CEO of a not-for-profit organization, notes that he worries about how a for-profit partner might use the organization's logo and brand. What risks is he considering?

2. Melia also suggests that not-for-profits get "wrapped up in their own principles" and thereby miss opportunities with the private sector and partnering. What does he mean?

3. Melia provides two great recommendations to a not-for-profit. Pick a not-for-profit organization that you know well and describe how those recommendations could help that organization in a partnership.

Conclusion

Chapter 8 introduces a number of specific tactics and strategies, as well as key concepts, for management and marketers of not-for-profit organizations in physical activity, sport participation, and public health to adopt to help their private-sector partners achieve their CSR objectives. A number of cases, Executive Perspectives, and content sections are provided. The cases offer examples and practices to follow, as do the contributions of industry experts. Further, the chapter provides a series of specific tactical recommendations, including stepwise directions for their use, that not-for-profit organizations can use. As noted earlier in the chapter, these tactics are especially useful for smaller not-for-profit organizations.

Putting Partnership Guidelines Into Action

Parts I and II of the book provided eight chapters of information, background, examples, and details on partnerships between the private sector and not-for-profit organizations in health, sport participation, and physical activity. Chapter 2 shares *The Partnership Protocol*, an industry-developed set of guidelines to develop and manage these partnerships in a responsible and effective way. The reality of these partnerships is then established in the remaining chapters, including tactical details of responsible management. A comprehensive view has been provided.

This leads us to part III, the final part of the book, which is meant to encourage the implementation of the various concepts and tactics. In this regard, three chapters are presented. Chapter 9 outlines the global, national, and community levels of partnerships in an effort to show how the perspective should be adopted in each of these three contexts. Chapter 10 follows with advice about applying *The Partnership Protocol*, using CATCH as a specific case example. Finally, chapter 11 outlines the challenges and other barriers that will need to be overcome to develop effective partnerships in the health, sport participation, and physical activity sectors.

PART

three

CHAPTER 9

Global, National, and Community Partnership Perspectives

Maybe it's time we apply the old idiom "Think globally, act locally" to sport and physical activity. Partnerships are increasingly going global as programs are delivered in multiple countries and regions, and immigration is diversifying communities culturally and ethnically. Reaching global, national, and community participants requires effective partnering across multiple sectors, using appropriate communication methods and platforms. Creating strong, legacy-building international and national events has long-term benefits in communities and surrounding regions. In varying scales of geographical focus, partnerships between public and private spheres have successfully developed world-class events, tournaments, products, and facilities that directly benefit local citizens in the regions that they touch.

Both public and private organizations can benefit from partnerships as they share resources, expertise, and work toward mutual goals. As organizations in various sectors work to increase health and sport participation, partnerships are logical options to drive initiatives forward. In this chapter, we explore partnership perspectives in various scopes. At the global level, partners go beyond their borders and engage in initiatives and programs that can benefit citizens in multiple countries and nations around the world and the broader international community. At the national level, partnerships use strategies that will reach across their own countries with the possibility of generating national support and pride. At the community level, local groups and citizens take active roles in leading partnerships that best suit their community needs and wants. Although perspectives and scopes of partnerships differ, we see a common thread of mutual trust, respect, and sharing of resources in successful partnerships.

Partnering Across Sectors

Because sport and physical activity participation is decreasing or stagnating in communities (Vail 2007) and youth (Tremblay et al. 2010), international, national, and community organizations and leaders must seek new ways to promote wellness, fitness, and healthy lifestyles. Organizations, both public and private, can look across multiple sectors to find partners that offer new resources and better access to the populations that they hope to serve. As the international sport and development organization Right To Play (2008a) noted, it is important to "engage as many sectors as possible in developing and implementing physical activity promotion strategies," including (a) the health sector, (b) the sport sector, (c) the education sector, (d) the media, (e) local governments, and finally (f) national financial and economic policy makers (p. 66). Accordingly, the health sector can use evidence to advocate, inform, and build integrated networks with public and policy makers regarding the health, social, and economic benefits and barriers of physical activity. The sport sector can facilitate the use of sport facilities, allocate funds, provide sport training, and promote physical activities to all people regardless of ethnicity, social class, gender, or disability. The education sector can make school space available for community physical activity, commit to physical activity in the school curriculum, and encourage universities and colleges to undertake data collection, research, evaluation, and training for strategies to increase physical activity levels and set physical activity and sport as a platform for public education and communication. Schools are also prime sites for the delivery of physical activity and sport programs aimed at school-age children, teachers, and coaches (Right To Play 2008b). The media can promote physical activity through programming, circulating positive messages, and educating journalists to be advocates for physical activity. Local governments can support legislation and policies that promote safe and accessible indoor and outdoor physical activity spaces and programs. Finally, national financial and economic policy makers can allocate resources and encourage investment from public and private sectors to support physical activity, sport, and other health promotion programs. Partnering across sectors can garner widespread support that can translate into successful partnerships at the global, national, and local levels.

Global Perspectives

To promote health and sport outside and across national borders and to reach communities and cultures different from your own, engaging in partnerships make sense. At the global level, networks of partners can help build national and community support for programs and initiatives and provide better access to local gatekeepers. The following section highlights three organizations that have extensive global partnerships, each using their international networks to meet their organization's specific sport, physical activity, and health objectives: the International Platform on Sport and Development, Right To Play, and Agita São Paulo–Agita Mundo.

International Platform on Sport and Development

The International Platform on Sport and Development is a partnership between numerous public and private organizations: the Australian Sports Commission (ASC), Canadian Heritage (PCH), the International Sport and Culture Association (ISCA), the Laureus Sport for Good Foundation, NCDO (Dutch National Committee for International Cooperation and Sustainable Development), Nike (Nike's role in public–private partnerships will be detailed further in an upcoming section), the Norwegian Olympic and Paralympic Committee and Confederation of Sports (NIF), the Swiss Agency for Development and Cooperation (SDC), and the Union of European Football Associations (UEFA). The platform serves as a knowledge hub to facilitate and advance partnerships across sectors and stakeholder groups, using sport to foster broader economic, social, and individual development (Sport and

Development 2009a). The platform allows open access for organizations to post information about their partnership's objectives, target groups, partners, region of operation, duration, and status (i.e., active or nonactive). Each organization provides a summary of their physical activity or sport project, lessons learned, and the way in which physical activity and sport are used to support the project. The Sport and Development Partnership Toolkit includes a list of public and private benefits for partnering, as well as detailed examples of sport partnerships with the private sector (e.g., the KNVB Football for Development program, which aims to build local capacity by educating youth leaders, coaches, referees, and administrators; and the SCORE Sports Coaches' OutReach programs, which use sport for skill building in youth in South Africa, Namibia, and Zambia). Currently, the International Platform on Sport and Development hosts over 300 physical activity and sport projects, implemented around the world through public and private partnerships at the global, national, and community levels.

Right To Play

The humanitarian organization Right To Play, along with its public (e.g., Canadian Heritage) and corporate partners (e.g., Adidas, Aegon) coordinates programs in 23 countries worldwide. Top athletes deliver sport programs in local communities to support peace, conflict resolution, basic education, child development, health promotion, disease prevention, and community development. For Right To Play, public partners such as NGOs, amateur sport organizations, and local grassroots organizations play critical roles in physical activity partnerships. The public partners are essential trusted and respected intermediaries between the private sector or government and the communities and people to ensure that programs are delivered to those that they aim to reach. Right To Play's partnerships can contribute to partnership advocacy, development, and implementation. At the global level, Right To Play partners with an international network of sport NGOs and organizations, Kicking AIDS Out, to promote the use of sport and physical activity programs to deliver HIV–AIDS education and life skill training (Kicking AIDS Out 2008). Right To Play's extensive and multipurpose global networks use sport to promote peace, community building, leadership, and other values in communities around the globe.

Agita São Paulo–Agita Mundo

From Brazil to the world, the Agita São Paulo–Agita Mundo partnership brings together governmental, nongovernmental, and private-sector organizations to promote physical activity and health among the population. Agita São Paulo is a partnership based on an ecological model; through a central organizing body it synchronizes three broad aspects: intrapersonal environment (e.g., demographics and behaviors), social environment (e.g., culture and governing structures), and physical environment (e.g., natural environment, facilities, transportation). The choice of the partnership name *Agita*, meaning "to agitate," aims to convey the goal of the partnership: to move Brazilians through both physical activity and social mobilization. As Matsudo and Matsudo (2006) noted, the Agita São Paulo partnership aimed to inspire "physical, mental and social movement towards an active citizenship" (p. 134). The partnership benefited from national and international "intellectual" partners, including national and international organizations that provided scientific, logistic, political, and administrative input, such as the U.S. Centers for Disease Control and Prevention (CDC), the International Union for Health Promotion and Education (IUHPE), the Dallas Aerobic Institute, and the World Health Organization (WHO). Locally, the program offered open, multisector partnerships to any organization who aimed to promote physical activity and wellness in São Paulo; the program then spread to national (Physical Activity Network of the Americas: RAFA-PANA) and international (Agita Mundo) networks (Matsudo and Matsudo 2006). The open membership empowered local organizations to use the partnership to meet the needs of their communities and groups in the best way. Agita Mundo currently hosts 236 member institutions in 58 countries.

Megaevents

Major international sporting events are most often the result of ambitious international partnerships. New sporting facilities are occasionally prompted by ambitions to bid for or host national and international events such as the Olympic Games, Commonwealth Games, World Cup, and other major sport championships. These megaevents, as described by Andranovich, Burbank, and Heying (2001), can stimulate economic growth and justify local spending and allocation of resources. Through successful megaevents, partnerships can have lasting influence by cultivating future tourism and spurring profitable development in the surrounding region.

Olympic Games

The Olympic Games unvaryingly bring the world's presence and attention to the host region. In the development of the Salt Lake City Games, the partnership involved private (entrepreneurial) funding in collaboration with Salt Lake City and the state of Utah. The formation of a not-for-profit group (Salt Lake City Olympic Organizing Committee, SLOC) aspired to reimage Utah as the winter sport capital of North America, generate state revenues of $900 million, and provide a lasting legacy for Utah (Andranovich, Burbank, and Heying 2001, p. 119). A 1989 public referendum, approved by 57 percent of state residents, diverted $59 million in sales tax revenue to fund the construction of Olympic facilities and lay the foundation for more aggressive bidding on the Games by the city. SLOC encouraged urban revitalization and development (e.g., airport improvements and development of a light rail line). But the role of local government and local citizens was unclear in the partnership agreement, leading to discord between public and private interests and resulting in doubtful economic viability of the facilities beyond the Olympic Games and an uncertain post-Olympic legacy.

In contrast, the Sydney Olympics, as described by Wettenhall (2003), was deemed a partnership success. It created a new model that the International Olympic Committee hoped would be adopted by other host countries. The federal and city governments formed the public side, and the International and Australian Olympic Committees made up the private side. The Sydney Organising Committee for the Olympic Games (SOCOG), created to provide public accountability, included representation from all partners. During the preparation period, the private partners controlled the bid for and the development of the Games, but as opening day approached, the New South Wales government strengthened its role. The government directed the 2000 Olympic Games' operation effectively and created a lasting legacy.

Homeless World Cup

A unique international sporting event that draws multisector partners is the Homeless World Cup, first held in 2003. The annual international soccer tournament unites over 25,000 homeless and excluded people who represent their countries, and it supports the development of grassroots soccer projects in more than 64 nations (Homeless World Cup 2009). With a long list of partners and major support from private companies (such as UEFA, Nike, UN, Manchester United, Real Madrid) and professional athletes, the event generates greater awareness of homelessness and exclusion and can inspire and motivate homeless people to better their lives through participation in sport. Benefits are reaped concurrently by players, local grassroots organizations, and the local and international communities.

National Perspectives

At the national level, partnerships can include national sport organizations, not-for-profits, and national government support. National partnerships can be part of the development of major national sport events (e.g., Canada Winter Games) or part of the creation of products or programs to be delivered to citizens across the country.

Healthy Kids Program

In Canada, the Healthy Kids program, led by *Today's Parent* magazine, created online tools and resources and uses the magazine articles and contests to promote education aimed at injury prevention, fitness and nutrition, mental health, and environment and health. National program partners include Safe Kids Canada (a national injury prevention program of the Hospital for Sick

Children), Boys and Girls Clubs of Canada, Kids Help Phone, Canadian Partnership for Children's Health & Environment, Arts for Children and Youth, YMCA, Canadian Women's Foundation, Girls' Growth Fund IPO (Immediate Public Opportunity), Fire Prevention Canada, Spark Together for Healthy Kids (a Heart and Stroke Foundation program), and At My Best (a school-based children's wellness program developed by AstraZeneca Canada and Physical and Health Education Canada) (*Today's Parent* 2009).

Canadian Multicultural Hockey Championship

As a national partnership, the Canadian Multicultural Hockey Championship, established in 2007, leverages its sport component to benefit local players, organizations, and communities. Under the leadership of OMNI Television executive producer Stanley Papulkas, partnerships were developed with sport and community organizations and hockey clubs with diverse ethnic groups in Toronto (CMHL 2009). The event quickly grew to 16 teams of culturally diverse Canadians. Players of ethnic descent from Italy, Ireland, China, Japan, Korea, Russia, Greece, Finland, Portugal, and other regions vied for the Canada Cup. The event led to the creation of the Canadian Multicultural Hockey League (CMHL), which brought together the Canadian Italian Hockey League and the Japanese Canadian Hockey League, and included the organizers of the Asian Hockey Tournament, a tournament that had been bringing together Asian Canadians for more than 15 years. Individual professional athletes who supported the event included former NHL players Peter Zezel (Serbian team), Nikolai Borschevsky (Russian team), and Mark Osborne (Ukrainian team and tournament spokesman). According to the CMHL (2009), the league is now open to both Canadian men and Canadian women. Among the 17 teams are the Scottish Marauders, Portuguese Sea Wolves, Polish Hussars, Ojibwe Thunderbirds, Chinese Ice Dragons, and the Estonians Ice. Also competing is a United World Team for Canadians from ethnic groups that are not formally represented in the league.

Creating National Products

Public and private partners align to cocreate products that are part of national injury prevention and sport and health promotion strategies. In Canada the Forzani Group (Sport Chek, Sport Mart, National Sports) partnered with Hockey Canada to produce *Hockey 101*, a free introductory hockey education booklet distributed nationally to parents with first-time children hockey players. The booklet includes information on rules, fair play, and required equipment (Forzani Group 2009). Another example is the ThinkFirst program series, a set of educational booklets and videos prepared by private partners (e.g., Intrawest Corporate) and national or provisional sport organizations or not-for-profit groups (e.g., Ronald McDonald House) to develop safety instruction and injury prevention for skiing, equestrian, hockey, and soccer

Partnership Highlight

A LOOK AT GLOBAL PARTNERSHIPS
IN ACTION: NIKE

Nike, as one of the world's largest designers, marketers, and distributors of sport and fitness footwear, apparel, equipment, and accessories (Nike 2004), takes on a significant role in partnering with public organizations to deliver sport and physical activity programs to generate a myriad of outcomes. Nike has a dedicated corporate responsibility platform and is committed to being a "responsible global citizen" and engaging with the world (Nike 2004). With partners including Right To Play and as an international member of the International Platform on Sport and Development, Nike is a major contributor to sport and physical activity programs that create opportunities for social inclusion, gender equality, peace, environmental awareness, and many other issues. Four of Nike's partnerships are worth highlighting: the Nike Foundation, Nike Changemakers, Nike CARE, and Nike Gamechangers.

■ Nike Foundation: Led by President Maria Eitel since 2004, the Nike Foundation invests in programs and mobilizes resources that focus on adolescent girls in the developing world (Nike 2008a). The foundation's investments are aimed toward gaps identified by current partners, usually directed through requests for proposals (RFPs) for girl-specific programming. Grants range from $10,000 to $1.5 million (Nike 2008a). The foundation partners in programs worldwide and has particular interest in Bangladesh, Brazil, China, Ethiopia, India, Kenya, Zambia, Uganda, and Liberia. According to the Nike Foundation's website (Nike 2008a), "Underlying every invitation, every proposal review and every grant agreement is our desire to learn, understand, nurture and share how to unleash girls' powerful ripple effect." The Nike Foundation partners with the International Center for Research on Women, Save the Children, the Massachusetts Institute of Technology Poverty Action Lab, and the Population Council to help measure the impact of their programs and establish a formula of success based on the lessons learned from the field. In 2005 the Nike Foundation along with the United Nations Foundation led a multisectored partnership called the Coalition for Adolescent Girls to mobilize support from corporate, religious, and cultural leaders to recognize the power of girls in addressing global health issues. A new program, the Girl Effect, aims to advocate for girls by "yelling from a virtual rooftop" to educate leaders about how the participation of girls can create conditions of social and economic change (Nike 2008a).

■ Nike Changemakers: In 2007 Nike partnered with Ashoka Changemakers to launch the Sport for a Better World competition. The competition aimed to allow collaborative, open, and interactive opportunities for individuals and organizations of a variety of sizes and goals to present proposals that would use sport and physical activity to transform lives and communities (Nike 2007). Sport for a Better World encouraged sport-based social entrepreneurship and drew 120 entries from 40 countries, including a Venezuelan proposal aiming to increase access and end corruption within municipal sport programs, a United States organization aiming to help youth in East Africa learn how to use their running skills to gain scholarships for education and make careers in sport, and an Egyptian project that uses a volleyball league to promote girls' rights to education and participation in school (Nike 2007). Winners earned $5,000 toward their programs. Applicants were judged by members of the National Basketball Association (NBA), International Olympic Committee, FC Barcelona, Nike, United Nations Children's Fund (UNICEF), and the founder of the Homeless World Cup.

■ Nike CARE: Nike's partnership with CARE (a U.S.-based humanitarian organization that fights global poverty) and the Mathare Youth Sports Association (MYSA) (a Kenyan youth organization that links sport with community service) connects sport with leadership training, AIDS prevention, cleanups, and other community service activities in one of Africa's poorest regions (Nike 2009). Through the partnership, "The MYSA soccer program offers players a high level of training and coaching, and some get international experience. The exhibition games in the U.S. are in part a showcase of their talents for college coaches and scouts" (Nike 2009). The program selects girls based on academic performance and community involvement, as well as athletic ability. The Nike CARE partnership with MYSA strives for gender equity because it empowers women, resolves conflict, and bridges cultural divides (Nike 2009).

■ Nike Gamechangers: Nike Gamechangers partner with numerous social change organizations around the world to promote sport as an agent of change. For instance, Nike and its partners in the Sport for Social Change Network (SSCN) (a network of 26 not-for-profits from across Brazil) converged to work toward ensuring that all children in São Paulo and across Brazil can access sport and find places to play (Nike 2008b). Nike (2008b) described Nike Gamechangers this way:

> It's not about one person. Or one company. Or one donation. It's about all of us. Working together. As a team. Because when we play together, the competition—global warming, HIV, poverty, inequality, despair—doesn't stand a chance. We've got the skills, the players, and the determination to go full out until we've beaten each and every thing standing between us and a world where any person, anywhere, can go outside and compete. The world is our playing field. So, let's go out there, beat anything and change everything.

Nike, through its various partnerships, has affirmed its commitment to corporate social responsibility by promoting and delivering programs that use sport and physical activity in disadvantaged communities and supporting local grassroots operations.

GLOBAL APPLICATION QUESTIONS

1. Nike has had many successes as well as some negatives in its history. Describe the Nike brand and image from the perspective of a not-for-profit. Is this an organization that not-for-profits would like to partner with? Why or why not?

2. Many organizations, like Nike, have foundations. These entities are separate but affiliated organizations (details vary by country) that have a charitable purpose. Research foundations in your country or region and describe how they differ from the parent for-profit organization.

3. Nike is known for its strategy to endorse many of the world's best athletes. How can these athletes enhance a public–private partnership?

(ThinkFirst 2009). The product of the partnership can benefit citizens nationally as well as reach local communities.

Community Perspectives

For private organizations, partnering with public sport organizations helps them understand the needs of the local community, including interests, demand forecasts, and expectations as well as diversity (e.g., cultural) and accessibility (e.g. wheelchair access) considerations. To reach the local community, the partnership needs to generate local excitement about the partnership's commitment, aims, and accomplishments. To do this, as Gilmore (2004) explained, partnerships must consider the cultural needs of the community to ensure that services and products are accessible and inclusive of minority populations and inspire volunteerism or participation in the local community.

The needs of the community can be explored through expert input and public consultation. To direct sport partnerships between the City of Toronto and teams in the American Hockey League, Farag and Brittain (2009) noted that using direct opinion surveys could have been valuable in confirming potential interest from the public. Further, Rosentraub and Swindell (2009) noted that before a partnership builds a new professional sport facility in a community, it should consider the number of large private companies in the area and determine whether they are willing to purchase luxury seating (e.g., corporate boxes). Assessing the needs of the public can inform and direct the actions of the partnership and better prepare the partners for associated risks.

Public organizations may seek private partnerships to increase their community profiles and attract more local funding, especially sport and physical activity organizations that face a steady decline in government funding (Misener and Doherty 2009). Crabbe (2000) described a successful community partnership program, the Leyton Orient Community Sports Programme (a not-for-profit charity in London, UK), that partnered with professional soccer teams to introduce socially excluded groups to community activities through a year-long sport program that included education, behavior modification, and rehabilitation as strategies to decrease drug use in the community.

The education sector is often a key partner in delivering community-based programs aimed at increasing physical activity and wellness of children and teenagers. Programs such as Healthy Kids, Healthy Schools in Houston, Texas, draw on partners and resources to "improve nutrition and physical activity opportunities through a communications campaign, delivering new healthy food options to kids, working with local businesses and retail stores to create a Healthy School Zone" (Healthy Kids, Healthy Schools 2009). The partnership includes 23 organizations from multiple sectors including the National Dairy Council, City of Houston, and the University of Texas. The program also included student input; more than two dozen students acted as equal partners in creating the vision of the Healthy Kids, Healthy Schools wellness program.

Community Sport and Recreation Facilities

Recent academic literature in the sport and physical activity partnership context is heavily weighted in the examination of public government (e.g., city) and private enterprise partnerships aimed at building and managing new sport and recreational facilities, such as arenas and stadiums (see Farag and Brittain 2009; Ferk and Ferk 2008; Kennedy and Rosentraub 2000; Rosentraub and Swindell 2009; Roy 2008; Schrerer and Sam 2008; Siegfried and Zimbalist 2000).

City officials consider partnering with private organizations to be able to reap the benefits of building new sport facilities, including encouraging pride and community spirit, stimulating economic development, and creating new regional recreation patterns (Kennedy and Rosentraub 2000; Roy 2008).

New facilities may be able to promote healthy lifestyles and bring new fitness activities to the community. But Kennedy and Rosentraub (2000), Roy (2008), and Siegfried and Zimbalist (2000) argued that new sport facilities may not, as cities presupposed, boost the region's economy, but instead amass financial risk for the host communities. Pointing to new facilities for professional sport teams (Major League Baseball, National Basketball Association, and National Football League), Kennedy and Rosentraub (2000) found that public subsidies provided the substantial portion of facility funding, upward of hundreds of millions of dollars (e.g., MLB's Seattle Mariners' new stadium received a $360 million public subsidy). More optimistically, Roy (2008) found that new facilities for minor-league teams (AAA, AA, A, and independent franchises) do expand markets in smaller regions and can generate positive outcomes and profit when marketers focus on both attracting and retaining fans.

In considering new facilities, communities may consider partnering with a private organization to attract new users or the ability to generate more profit. Vining and Boardman (2008) proposed that users may be more willing to pay user fees for services that are offered by private operators as opposed to public operators (e.g., users would be willing to pay registration fees for privately operated sport facilities but expect city-run facilities to be free or low cost). If this rationale is accurate, arenas, ski hills, and other leisure facilities built through partnerships offer the opportunity to generate more revenue through participation fees.

At the community level, facilities usually include some balance between private and public input, funding, construction, land, and operating structures. Cities and municipalities can rarely be excluded from consideration when building a new facility. For instance, a new arena may require adjustments in traffic control patterns and new commitments in public safety expenditures (Rosentraub and Swindell 2009). In the case of the Cranbrook Civic Arena

Finding Consensus
in How to Develop Partnerships

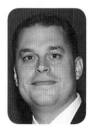

John-Paul Cody-Cox
Chief Executive Officer, Speed Skating Canada

BIO

John-Paul Cody-Cox has had a diversified career working in high tech, government, consulting, and ultimately in sport management for the last seven years. He is now chief executive officer of Speed Skating Canada, Canada's most successful Olympic sport.

Before taking his position as CEO of Speed Skating Canada, Cody-Cox was executive director of Volleyball Canada, where he led efforts to eliminate $1.7 million in debt in less than two years and simultaneously led a group of national sport organizations in generating $6 million in new funding for team sports. As director of marketing and sponsorships for Volleyball Canada, he oversaw its major event and sponsorship portfolio, increasing marketing and sponsorship revenues from $50,000 annually to $500,000. Before working at Volleyball Canada, Cody-Cox ran his own consulting firm, Momentum Sponsorship Strategies, worked as a program officer at Sport Canada, and was director of sponsorships and marketing programs for Corel Corporation, where he managed all sponsorship and corporate marketing programs, and oversaw various partnerships including the Ottawa Senators Hockey Club and Corel Centre, the Art Institutes, Sony, and Intel.

A native of Halifax, Nova Scotia, John-Paul attended Carleton University for his undergraduate studies in political science. After completing his undergraduate work, he earned his master's in political psychology at Wilfrid Laurier University and followed that up a few years later with his MBA from the University of Ottawa.

MY VIEW ON PARTNERSHIPS

Mandates should drive partnerships by finding like-minded groups in cities, governments, and communities. Too often partnerships miss prioritization of a match of values. Speed Skating Canada's partnership with Intact was based on mutual values of respect for people and sustainability to create proactive grassroots programs that meet business and values-based objectives.

PARTNERSHIPS IN ACTION:
VOLLEYBALL CANADA AND DOWNSVIEW PARK

Volleyball Canada's growth was fostered by appreciating business opportunities. To overcome the existing model of prioritizing national team beach programs and a shoe-string budget that was mostly devoted to staff salaries and training, Volleyball Canada had to consider business opportunities to grow the sport. The Pan Am Games offered an opportunity to develop a partnership with Downsview Park to create a national beach volleyball training center. Both partners invested in the project, which was built around each partner's specific mandate and principles and with support from community and national groups. Like a business, the partnership needed to make money, but the partnership was grounded in each partner's goals and values (without overestimating each partner's commitment and capacity). Each partner had different goals; Downsview aimed to bring more people in to the venue through increased participation and new opportunities to host events; Volleyball Canada saw the partnership as good for the sport in terms of increased access and promotion. Often, people don't take the time to make the call and ask, "Can we talk?" Downsview, with its rundown courts, may not have seemed like an obvious choice for partnership, but by calling, Volleyball Canada realized an opportunity to convert other underused space into a major volleyball center. The next step was to reach out beyond the partnership and consider who else in the community could help fund the proposed project. They were successful in securing a Trillium grant and obtaining support from Canadian Sport Centre Ontario for low-cost opportunities to add national-level coaching and administrative support. The Trillium grant acts as a buffer to develop a self-sufficient funding model.

LEVERAGING RECOGNITION: SPEED SKATING CANADA

Turning to Speed Skating Canada, John-Paul noted its strong brand recognition, amplified by the success of Canadian speed skaters in the Olympics. An attempt to leverage the recognition translated into developing community partnerships. In Halifax, a temporary speed skating oval that was created for the Canada Games was embraced by the community. A resulting "Save the oval" mission was pursued by a variety of stakeholders, who formed a loose partnership among media, government, city officials, community groups, and local citizens. With national-level support from Speed Skating Canada, ParticipACTION, Canadian Sport Centre Atlantic, and Canada Games, the oval was promoted as a venue for increasing community participation in recreational and high-level programs. Money for creating new infrastructure is often limited, but driven by community support and partnerships, the idea to save the existing oval was a realistic option. Making the oval a permanent facility in Halifax offers an example for future Canada Games planning. The question becomes, "How do we work to make this happen in every community?"

EMBRACING THE TREND TOWARD PARTNERSHIPS

The trend is moving to partnered approaches and away from the spirit of competition for members or participants. One of the challenges is that often sport organizations do not look at the system as a whole and instead focus on community-level or high-performance sport, and they fail to examine how community-level activity is a pipeline to greater overall membership. Sport Canada can do a better job of encouraging sport organizations to work better together. Again, a business approach should be taken by examining opportunities and looking at ways to decrease frustrations, gaps, and obstacles. The idea is to consider how organizations can work together and build from each other's capacity rather than build from scratch.

(continued) ▶

(continued) ▶

Curling is a good model of self-sufficiency in an ice sport; only 30 percent of funding comes from government, compared with the 70 to 85 percent that government contributes to speed skating. Government funding is difficult to manage and needs to be spent in a certain way. Accountability limits some self-directed growth strategies. The Canadian Team Sports Coalition was able to persuade government to invest an additional $6 million of funding into team sports through these multiple sports coming together. Within the coalition, separate entities of summer and winter sport groups came together to share resources and create strategic relations. No individual sport would have been able to achieve its goal alone. Together and focused, the coalition demonstrates the power of partnership.

GLOBAL APPLICATION QUESTIONS

1. A national sport organization (NSO) like Speed Skating Canada is a not-for-profit with a cause. But many people view the cause of high-performance sport as less important than things like cancer or AIDS or diabetes. Discuss this point and suggest how an NSO in your country could attract private-sector partners.

2. As a CEO at various not-for-profit organizations in his career, Cody-Cox has prioritized partnerships with the private sector. How important is it, in your view, for the leader of the not-for-profit to have such a focus?

3. In what cases would you suggest that partnerships with the private sector might not be appropriate for a not-for-profit sport organization?

Multiplex, as described by Vining and Boardman (2008), a public referendum voted in favor of a 30-year partnership that included the designing, building, and operating of the arena by Vestar Inc., partnered with the City of Cranbrook (British Columbia). In the mid-1990s, the private partner assumed operating risks of $1.5 million and capital cost of $22.6 million, and the public partner leased the land for the hockey arena, swimming pool, and other recreational facilities. The city was allocated 1,500 hours of facility time, and Vestar was able to generate revenues by selling the rest of the hours for recreational activities, special events, and concerts. The project was fraught with legal disputes, delays, and cost overruns, which resulted in new city taxes and eventually the termination of the partnership only 5 years into the 30-year agreement. Cranbrook developed the highest debt level of all municipalities in British Columbia (Vining and Boardman 2008). This case is an example of the consequences of a partnership that did not effectively consider the risks involved.

Charity Runs

Community walking and running events are good methods of raising awareness and generating support for a cause while providing opportunities for citizens to participate in physical activity in their community. Participants often run

Community Partnership Perspectives

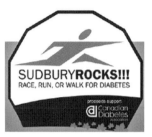

Jennifer MacKinnon
Regional Director (North East Ontario), Canadian
Diabetes Association

Vince Perdue
President Sudbury ROCKS!!! Running Club and Race
Director, Sudbury ROCKS!!! Race Run Walk for Diabetes

Sudbury, Ontario, Canada

Reprinted, by permission, from
Sudbury.

BUILDING PARTNERSHIPS FROM COMMON MISSIONS

Across the country, the Canadian Diabetes Association (CDA) is leading the fight against diabetes by helping people with diabetes live healthy lives while we work to find a cure. We are supported in our efforts by a community-based network of volunteers, members, employees, health care professionals, researchers, and partners. By providing education and services, advocating on behalf of people with diabetes, supporting research, and translating research into practical applications, we are delivering on our mission. The CDA builds services around the needs of people with diabetes in the local community, helping them stay healthy while also paying careful attention to donors and donor wishes. The Sudbury ROCKS!!! Running Club's mission shares CDA's value placed on healthy living and broadens it to encourage and support the development of public participation in running for fitness, health, and enjoyment. Both organizations work with private and public partners and individual supporters to help contribute to our missions.

PARTNERSHIPS IN ACTION: THE SUDBURY ROCKS!!! RACE RUN WALK FOR DIABETES

The Sudbury ROCKS!!! Race Run Walk for Diabetes evolved from a series of smaller Sun Runs that were part of the Sudbury Fitness Challenge (in Sudbury, Ontario, Canada). A partnership between the CDA and the Sudbury ROCKS!!! Running Club, driven by a community leader who moved in a "go big or go home" style, envisioned the race as a way to get the community rallying around physical activity and health. The CDA was a natural partner because Sudbury ROCKS!!! club members had previously taken part in CDA's national fund-raising programs by participating in overseas marathons with Team Diabetes. With the increased reach and profile that the partnership with CDA offered, the running event grew from 150 participants in the Sun Run, to 450 participants in the first year of the Sudbury ROCKS!!! Race Run Walk for Diabetes events, to more than 2,000 participants five years later in 1K, 5K, 10K, half marathon, marathon, team relay, and celebrity and mascot challenge events. To reciprocate for being selected as the recipient charity for runner pledges, the CDA offered administrative support and a presence on the race-planning executive team. The CDA also hosts a Northern Ontario Heritage–funded employee who works full time on developing and promoting the partnership event.

(continued) ▶

(continued) ▶

Our partnership was created out of a desire to fight the perception that we were a "fat city" and to create a showcase event that was in the faces of Sudburians and on the streets of Sudbury. We didn't want to change just fitness levels; we also wanted to change the perceptions of health and fitness in our community. First, people would start to see us on the streets. The next year they might start cheering us on as we passed by their lawns, and then they might decide to participate. We always wanted kids involved; by making the Kids 1K a free event, we bring out parents to the race, and we've started to see generation building as parents and other family members start to get involved.

Both private and public donors offer title sponsorship (e.g., Ross Insurance Group Eight-Person Marathon Relay and the YMCA Strong Kids 1K), and local and regional businesses support several other levels of sponsorship. Many of the event's sponsors are related to the running community (e.g., employees or owners who are members and friends of the Sudbury ROCKS!!! Running Club). The CDA does 90 percent of the promotion work with smaller donors and finalizing contracts, while the Sudbury ROCKS!!! Running Club helps to seek major corporate sponsors. Along with the support of the CDA, a strong event champion in the leadership of Sudbury ROCKS!!! Running Club president Vince Perdue drives new partnerships and attracts sponsors.

RUNNING TO SUCCESS

The Sudbury ROCKS!!! Race Run Walk for Diabetes meets CDA's objective of promoting exercise, which is one of the pillars of type 2 diabetes prevention and preventing the secondary complications of all types of diabetes. Through the event, the CDA is also able to raise awareness of the signs and symptoms of prediabetes. Distinctly, one of the goals from the perspective of the Sudbury ROCKS!!! Running Club is to provide a highly competitive and well-organized training and race experience for runners. The dissimilarity in these goals does pose a marketing challenge because the CDA's event focus is on delivering a charitable fund-raising and community health promotion opportunity, whereas the ROCKS!!! partners want to market the race as the best running event in Northern Ontario and aim to reach runners beyond the Greater Sudbury community. Despite the divergent goals, as partners we had parallel visions in increasing community health and fitness participation and perceptions. We were successful at bringing increased awareness of diabetes to target populations and related diabetes partners and supporters (e.g., the Diabetes Education and Care Program, and the Sudbury Regional Hospital team) while also offering a showcase running event promoted within running clubs, fitness magazines, and websites throughout the province (and growing nationally).

We are pleased that almost everyone in Northern Ontario knows what the Sudbury ROCKS!!! Race Run Walk for Diabetes is. Our media support has been phenomenal; a CBC Radio running club invited community members to participate in weekly runs with radio hosts and showcased running topics (and free event promotion) in regular weekly segments. Other Celebrity Challenge participants from newsprint, TV, and radio talked up the event and their own participation leading up to race day. We also created an annual scholarship for a student race participant or volunteer who contributed to healthy living and diabetes awareness; the scholarship helped us attract, and give back to, more young people in our community.

We are proud of the growth of the Sudbury ROCKS!!! Race Run Walk for Diabetes. Smaller races are now looking to us and trying to emulate our success (e.g., Run for Patrick in North Bay, Ontario). We are always looking for ways to improve. One of the hardest things is to develop and maintain a solid working race committee. The commitment can be stressful, and volunteers devote countless hours, so we really need to work with people who share our passion. We needed a few years to establish a committee that effectively shared responsibilities and that we could trust to move our goals forward. Our volunteer committee works with a rotating leader, an approach that helps us avoid burnout and keep good people engaged.

The CDA's partnership with the Sudbury ROCKS!!! Running Club, with the support of community organizations, business groups, and individuals, has placed the Sudbury ROCKS!!! Race Run Walk for Diabetes as a long-term fixture in the community, an event that extends benefits in diabetes prevention, awareness, and education, and broader health and fitness promotion in community. It's a partnership that makes sense in the long run.

ADVICE: RUNNING A SMOOTH PARTNERSHIP

1. You need to believe in your partners. Many good causes are out there, but the closer to home the values are, the more sense the partnership makes. Motivation and passions need to move in the same direction and be more than just a professional or money-driven relationship. Both partners commit more than just resources. The partnership and outcomes rely on personal commitment, time, and energy to drive it forward.

2. Draw on each other's horsepower and strongest assets. If you can engage your partner to help you in every way possible, then you reduce the likelihood that one partner will burn out or leave the partnership. Having this mutual commitment is imperative to maximize each other's strengths.

It is important to recognize the value of a partnership leader and champion (like our race director, Vince Perdue). Partnerships need someone who walks the walk with 100 percent commitment and sets high standards that can draw new participants, volunteers, sponsors, and media interest.

GLOBAL APPLICATION QUESTIONS

1. In general, why would a major charity like the Canadian Diabetes Association partner with a local run like Sudbury ROCKS?

2. As a participant in the run, would it matter to you whether the club running the event (Sudbury ROCKS) was for-profit or not-for-profit? Would that issue matter to you if you were a donor?

3. One of the sponsors of a subevent (i.e., the Ross Insurance Group Eight-Person Marathon Relay) is a for-profit partner, and another (i.e., the YMCA Strong Kids 1K) is a not-for-profit. Do you notice a difference? Would it matter if the Ross Insurance Group sponsored the kids 1K run?

Participant as Partner:
A Participant Shares Her Story

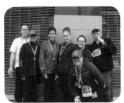

© Tammy Belanger

Tammy Belanger

Mid-30s, Type 1 Diabetes

Sudbury ROCKS!!! Race Run Walk for Diabetes Participant

PARTNERSHIPS IN ACTION: A PARTICIPANT'S PER-SPECTIVE

Last year, my colleague approached me about participating in the Sudbury ROCKS!!! Race Run Walk for Diabetes, a local running event in our community. The event is a partnership between Sudbury ROCKS!!! Running Club and the Canadian Diabetes Association. Financial support is provided by local business, community, and media sponsors. At the time I laughed; I am so not a runner. But the cause was close to my heart (I have type 1 diabetes), and it was just for fun, so I agreed to participate in the race as one of eight members of a marathon relay team. I had tried to find other events in our community that supported diabetes and did participate in a walk for the Juvenile Diabetes Research Foundation, but it was all kids and I felt completely out of place even though it was a smaller event.

As soon as I agreed to do the ROCKS!!! race, we started a four-week training program. I had done absolutely no running before. My first experience in the race was fun; it rained but we still had so much fun. We did it as a team, so we would cheer on each person as they ran to the next relay station. I saw the race as a way to support diabetes by raising money and having fun in the city at the same time. As a team we raised pledges and talked about our upcoming race; I raised $200 that first year. At the end of the race, we were pumped! We went for a drink and decided right away that we would participate again next year. We started planning to meet for group training runs, usually once or twice per week. All of a sudden, I started to really enjoy running.

We participated in our second race this year. We made T-shirts and collected more pledges. Physically, I started to see a difference in myself. I lost weight, and running gave me the perspective that "I can do it too." I have type 1 diabetes, and I'll always require insulin, but with running I've started to adjust my intake levels because at times when I exercise I require less insulin. I also started to realize that there were all these people around me who were running who were just like me. I had always had a vision in my mind of what a runner should look like, but at the event you see all different shapes and sizes. It's really cool. It's motivating to see all the other people doing it.

I'm now getting more people involved, including my sisters and friends. It's nice to have supportive people around you. I think when people hear 5K, they don't realize how long it is. I was telling my parents about the route for my 5K practice race, and my mom couldn't believe how far I could run. I was proud that I could do it. I've already started planning for next time—I am hoping to run a 10K next year!

GLOBAL APPLICATION QUESTIONS

1. Do you see value in getting the perspective of participants (like Belanger) in an event? Why or why not?

2. Belanger notes that she planned to return to the event the following year and to encourage friends and family to do so as well. This outcome is extremely positive. In general, what can you do to encourage and maximize word of mouth?

3. How would you recommend the event respond if Belanger's account of her experience had been negative?

for a cause by collecting pledges or donating participation fees to the associated local or national charity. Charity runs are often led by organizations with the support of corporate private sponsors and the efforts of countless individual volunteers.

Charity runs can be a substantial source of revenue and promotion for the charity, but another important consideration is the impact of charity runs in promoting physical activity among participants. See the Executive Perspective in this chapter in which a diabetic participant in the Sudbury ROCKS!!! Race Run Walk for Diabetes shares her important perspective of a partnership.

Conclusion

Putting partnership guidelines in action, and for action, requires partnering across various sectors. Organizations, both public and private, operate on various global, national, and community scales depending on their intended goals, but the common thread is the necessary partnering that helps link organizations to the populations that they attempt to serve. In this chapter, we examine diverse partnership perspectives and examples of successful partnerships that address international, national, and local needs. As we move forward to the coming chapters, you should consider your own organization's scope and objectives. Where do you fit, and how are you interacting with important local partners that help you reach your target group? Partnership perspectives are as different as the partnerships themselves. Success comes from recognizing unique partner strengths and listening carefully to the needs and wants of citizens in the local community.

Applying Partnership Guidelines in Physical Activity and Health

The first nine chapters of the book have laid out the key aspects, challenges, barriers, and tactical elements in the management of partnerships between the public sector and the private sector in the domains of sport participation, physical activity, and health. Most important, the guidelines have been explained, supported, and presented in detail. If the book has accomplished its purpose, you are now considering the use of the guidelines in prospecting, building, managing, and evaluating your partnerships. To arm you to complete these tasks, this chapter provides examples of how the guidelines can work in specific organizations.

This chapter presents case studies that illustrate partnerships between the public sector and the private sector in sport participation, physical activity, and health. The chapter includes one detailed case study and examples of other cases. The first part of the chapter is a case study, supported by the input of an industry expert, that outlines the successful partnership initiatives of a group of organizations working in the area of child health in the United States. The second part of the chapter includes mini-case-study examples, including a Canadian example built from publicly available information that outlines a recent partnership that is valuable to both the public- and private-sector partners. A table of examples of related partnerships is also included.

CATCH Case Study

The Coordinated Approach to Child Health, or CATCH, is a successful and established program founded by the University of Texas as part of a study funded by the National Heart, Lung, and Blood Institute in the early 1990s. That study assessed the effectiveness of school physical education and health education. Led by researchers from the University of Texas, Tulane University, the University of Minnesota, and the University of California at San Diego, the study provided the starting point for the establishment of a research center and a program dedicated to children's health. Figure 10.1 is a photo of 4 kids participating in CATCH.

The groundwork, including the initial concept and related research basis, that led to the development of CATCH started at the University of Texas in 1988, and the program gained traction by 1998. Today, CATCH continues to be managed by the University of Texas, and it has evolved to become what many consider the most coordinated and comprehen-

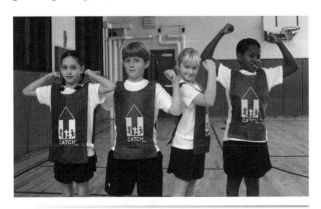

FIGURE 10.1 **Growing strong through CATCH school-based health, sport, and nutrition initiatives.**

Photo courtesy of CATCH®.

sive school-based health initiative in North America. Its success, as described by a long-time consultant with CATCH, Steve Lusk, is based on its approach to program development, which is evidence based, outcome focused, and stakeholder driven (i.e., involving parents, teachers, nutritionists, school administrators, and community partners). The program's accolades are extensive. More than 90 research papers have been published on its impacts. It received an award in 2012 from the Centers for Disease Control, and the Public Health Agency of Canada citation as a Best Practice for Health Promotion.

The CATCH office is located on the campus of the University of Texas within the Michael & Susan Dell Center for the Advancement of Healthy Living (Dell Center) in the University of Texas School of Public Health. The Dell Center, managed by two of the original CATCH researchers, supports and manages the CATCH program. Currently, the center has 28 staff and 21 professors who contribute to its research efforts. The work of the research teams at the University of Texas involves reviewing, evaluating, and developing aspects of CATCH to enhance its effectiveness as a program. They seek to make CATCH more efficient and sustainable. As part of this work, the researchers in the Dell Center develop content and train instructors for the program.

Currently, the CATCH program is composed of a learning pedagogy (i.e., curriculum) for kindergarten to eighth grade that includes, among a number of valuable tools, physical activity boxes, nutrition guides, an after-school program, a camp program, early childhood curriculum, information on diabetes prevention, tobacco avoidance planning, recommendations for reduced TV watching, healthy eating guides, and specific lessons for both gardening and physical activity. Figures 10.1, 10.2, and 10.3 are photos of CATCH participants in action.

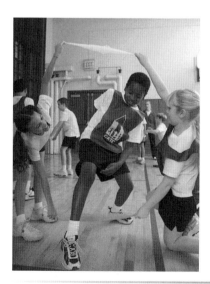

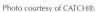

FIGURE 10.2 **CATCH kids in action, from kindergarten to grade 8.**

Photo courtesy of CATCH®.

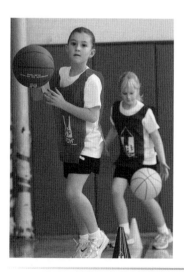

FIGURE 10.3 **Building healthy habits: Participants maintain more physical activity in their lives after the CATCH intervention program.**

Photo courtesy of CATCH®.

Evidence

CATCH, by most metrics, has been a successful program in making a difference in pursuit of its objectives. It began in 1991 as a randomized controlled community trial in 96 schools broken down into two groups of 56 (intervention) and 40 (control), and in 1994 expanded to four sites in the United States funded through the National Heart, Lung, and Blood Institute and supervised by five academics from universities across the United States. At the time, CATCH was arguably the largest school-based health promotion study in the United States. It was funded by four different National Institutes of Health (NIH) grants. Following the trials, CATCH was shown to effect change in dietary and physical activity behaviors. The students who had been exposed to the intervention consumed less fat and participated in more physical activity outside of school. As a result, school cafeterias provided meals that were lower in fat, and students were more physically active during physical education classes. A follow-up study found that the changes in diet and physical activity were maintained three years postintervention. In addition, evaluations, frameworks, models, and additional tests were carried out. These resulted in numerous publications in scientific journals and much better knowledge about this group. One of the grants led to the implementation of the CATCH program in 2,500 Texas elementary schools. Recently, in March 2012, CATCH was selected by the Children's Center in Florida as part of the overall wellness program plan for children. In May 2012 the CATCH program was awarded a Pioneering Innovation Award for Systems Change in Texas.

Since 1997 CATCH researchers in Texas have generated approximately US$11 million in funding from public and private sources. Similarly, more than US$5 million has been raised in New Mexico. Topics of research have been extensive and have included determining optimum training strategies, parent and community involvement, continuing education, curriculum development, communications message development, coalition building, and social networking. CATCH also emphasizes a coordinated and standardized approach that sees its programs seeking to align parents, teachers, nutritionists, school staff, and other partners in teaching healthy lifelong physical activity and diet behaviors. Texas is the site of CATCH's greatest success; more than 2,500 (or 50 percent) of the state's elementary schools adopt and use the program.

With respect to the program objective of reducing childhood obesity, CATCH has achieved some documented successes. First, an evaluation study done in El Paso found significant effects on the prevention of the onset of overweight and obesity among children when CATCH is implemented. Specifically, the study noted that following three years of CATCH implementation, in the intervention group 11 percent fewer girls and 9 percent fewer boys were classified as at risk to become overweight. Second, researchers in Texas undertook a cost-effectiveness study of CATCH and reported the program to be an excellent public investment. They found a cost-effectiveness benefit of $889.68 and a net benefit of $68,125—both numbers based on a comparison of the present value of averted (due to CATCH) future costs. Third, the School Physical Activity and Nutrition (SPAN) study compared students in grades 4, 8, and 11 in Texas using a large-population sample and found a statewide leveling off in the prevalence of overweight in children in the state at all grade levels and in all regions of Texas. More important, among 4th graders and 11th graders (largely Hispanic), a 7 percent reduction in the prevalence of overweight youth was found.

The Partnership

In 1998 the University of Texas entered into a partnership with FlagHouse Inc., a publishing and distribution firm, to manage the CATCH program. The rationale for the partnership was the interest of the University of Texas in maximizing the dissemination of its work and research. Management of the CATCH program felt that communication of the university's work and efforts was lacking, so they decided to explore options to improve this situation. The option of a partnership with an organization with expertise in providing such a service was considered, and a relationship with FlagHouse developed.

FlagHouse is a premier global publisher and supplier of resources for physical activity, recreation, education, and special needs. With operations in the United States and Canada, the for-profit organization's mission is to enhance the quality of life for people of all ages and abilities. It offers more than 20,000 innovative, high-quality products and resources. FlagHouse has served public- and private-sector customers for more than 50 years, including schools, parks, community centers, health care and treatment centers, and military bases. The organization's brands and catalogs include FlagHouse PE & Rec (Physical Education and Recreation), CATCH (Coordinated Approach to Child Health), Flying Start (for early childhood), Giant Leap (for children with special needs), and Going Strong (for adults with special needs). FlagHouse is a family-owned and operated for-profit company and employs well over 100 people.

Partnerships are a key element of the FlagHouse strategy, and the organization has partnered with a number of other not-for-profits:

- Project Adventure, the leader in experiential and adventure education programming in the United States
- YMCA of the USA
- YMCA Canada

- Boys and Girls Clubs of America
- Boys and Girls Clubs of Canada
- American Alliance for Health, Physical Education, Recreation and Dance
- National Association for Sport and Physical Education
- American Association for Physical Activity and Recreation
- Special Olympics USA
- Special Olympics Canada

For a current list of partners, see www.flaghouse.com/Athletic-partners. asp. Normally, in its partnerships, FlagHouse is involved in providing the overall responsibility for every facet of their commitment to their partners.

FlagHouse is based in New Jersey and has 5 staff dedicated to work nationally (United States) on the CATCH program. In Canada, FlagHouse has 30 full-time staff, one of whom is dedicated to CATCH. Collectively, the CATCH team at FlagHouse is highly experienced (more than 50 years of combined physical education and CATCH experience). This team provides technical assistance, supports implementation at schools, manages training on the CATCH Program, and leads the CATCH website www.catchinfo.org and monthly CATCH newsletter.

Components of the CATCH Partnership

The partnership between the University of Texas and FlagHouse is highly involved, and both partners describe CATCH as successful. Lusk describes the relationship as a "true partnership." The University of Texas develops and approves all content. In turn, FlagHouse distributes it and markets it, acting much like a publisher by offering a variety of services, including contract and project management, fulfillment of materials and equipment, and all billings. They also schedule and coordinate training of instructors. FlagHouse currently has contracts in place with a number of CATCH program partners, and the partners have agreed not to enter into any other contracts required for the provision of the requested services.

Through the course of the history of the partnership, the CATCH program has received state, national, and international recognition for being one of the most comprehensive and ambitious approaches to targeting physical education, food services, classroom curriculum, and families through a coordinated school health program. Such awards include the United States

Department of Health and Human Services Secretary's Innovation in Prevention Award in 2006 and the President's Council on Physical Fitness and Sport 2006 President's Challenge Active Lifestyle Award. The program has been recognized by many organizations for its effectiveness, including the School of Public Health at the University of North Carolina at Chapel Hill, HSC Foundation, Alliance for a Healthier Generation, Canadian Best Practices Portal for Health Promotion and Chronic Disease Prevention, Institute of Medicine, National Concern Institute, National Governor's Association, National Institute of Medicine, National Institute of Health, American Council for Fitness and Nutrition, Active Healthy Kids Canada, and many more. A subcomponent is the CATCH Kids Club, which has also been recognized broadly, won awards, and attracted grants to support its implementation.

As defined, CATCH is a program designed to promote physical activity, encourage healthy food choices, and prevent tobacco use in elementary-school-aged children. The program employs a holistic approach to child health promotion by targeting multiple aspects of the school environment and involving classroom teachers, school food service staff, physical education (PE) teachers, students' families, and the broader school community in a range of health-promoting activities for all school-aged children. The four core components of CATCH include (a) the Eat Smart school cafeteria nutrition program, (b) physical activity and healthy eating classroom curricula, (c) the CATCH physical education program, and (d) a family education and involvement program. The coordination of health messages and activities between these four component areas is critical to having a positive effect on children's knowledge, skills, and behavior.

In October 2011 the University of Texas and FlagHouse partnered with the Jared Foundation around the CATCH program in which the foundation (founded by the spokesman for Subway restaurants) endorsed CATCH as its official child wellness program. The three organizations (University of Texas, FlagHouse, Jared Foundation) partnered to continue their respective and collaborative efforts toward reducing childhood obesity. This arrangement is an example of extending a partnership to include an additional partner to expand its benefits further.

CATCH and *The Partnership Protocol*

Table 10.1 summarizes the links in the partnership between the University of Texas and FlagHouse around CATCH and some of the key elements of *The Partnership Protocol*.

TABLE 10.1   Applying *The Partnership Protocol*

Select elements in *The Partnership Protocol*	Details in the University of Texas–FlagHouse Partnership CATCH
Mutually beneficial outcomes for partners	Improved child welfare, reduced childhood obesity, business for FlagHouse.
Scarcity of government resources	No core government funding for CATCH program.
Escalating competition for resources	Varied sources of funding for CATCH since 1997.
Definition of a partnership	Fits precisely—the University of Texas as a not-for-profit health organization and FlagHouse as a for-profit partner.
Strength of partnership	The University of Texas and FlagHouse have been partners for many years, supporting each other's achievement of their own objectives.
Share each other's equity	The CATCH program shares in FlagHouse's ability to get their story out, create awareness, and provide distribution. FlagHouse shares in CATCH's successes in making a difference for its cause.
Stay true to who you are	Strong match between partners that has lasted for many years without major incident or problem in this regard.
Acknowledge and manage risk	Both partners work well to make sure that CATCH gets attention.
Create compelling communications	This element is FlagHouse's expertise.
Inspire, motivate, and activate your stakeholders	This element is FlagHouse's expertise.
Be clear	Over its history, the partnership has stayed focused on its mission to improve child welfare and decrease childhood obesity.
Measure and evaluate	Multiple evaluations and studies show the effectiveness of the CATCH program.
Assessing potential partners	Initially, the University of Texas sought a partner for CATCH who could help them tell their story in a broad, far-reaching way. After an extensive search, FlagHouse was found to be the ideal fit.
Flexible, open communications approach	Both partners use such a philosophy.
Building partnerships and the relationship between the partners	Both partners have been focused on making this a mutually beneficial, long-term partnership.
Manage the relationship in a way that the public will understand and communicate it effectively to your wider audience	This element has been the focus of the partnership since day 1.
Create a clear and fair agreement or contract	Done.
Project management	Both partners have plans to maximize the benefits and effectiveness of the partnership, including initiation, definition, planning, execution, and termination.

The Inside View on the CATCH Partnership

Steve Lusk
Canadian Professional Sales Association
Consultant, FlagHouse

BIO

Steve Lusk, an active member of the Canadian Professional Sales Association, is a graduate of Ryerson University and lives in Toronto, Ontario. He is a highly motivated and passionate business professional who possesses considerable experience in implementing and overseeing sales programs, metrics, and goals. Currently, Lusk is the business development consultant for CATCH in Canada working for FlagHouse. Before joining the CATCH program, Lusk held a variety of progressive entrepreneurial, sales management, and sales positions with a number of Ontario-based organizations, including Holland Imports, Water Creations, Nursery Pro, Fabco Data, and Corporate Express.

MY VIEW ON PARTNERSHIPS

The partnership between the University of Texas and FlagHouse with the CATCH program has been, in my view, a great example of a successful public–private partnership and one that illustrates very well the usefulness and worth of *The Partnership Protocol*. As outlined in table 10.1, the partnership fits with each stage and substage of *The Partnership Protocol* and illustrates how the protocol can work and how partnerships can benefit and prosper from such an approach.

Specifically, for me the key element is the research and evidence that supports the efficacy of the program in reducing childhood obesity. The vast variety, flexibility, and range of resources available to participants, family, instructors, teachers, and administration stand the program apart from anything else currently available. The CATCH program is really a combination of many levels, types, and iterations of programs, including an after-school program, an early childhood component, adapted activities for children with special needs, and, of course, the school curriculum for grades K through 8. Further, CATCH includes the delivery of a complete turnkey program including its coordination and management through FlagHouse, who specializes in providing a complete package of curriculum and the equipment needed to facilitate the program. An example of one of these valuable tools is the Coordination Tool Kit, our published tool to support program management. Created by the CATCH team, this is an example of a private-sector partner providing its expertise to its public-sector partner for the overall benefit of the partnership. A copy of one of the elements of this toolkit is provided here.

The purpose of CATCH is to bring the school, community, and parents together to go in the same direction to build healthy kids in healthy schools. CATCH is broken into six categories: principals and administrators, classroom teachers, child nutrition, physical education, parent leaders, and specialized support

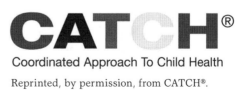

Reprinted, by permission, from CATCH®.

(continued) ▶

(continued) ▶

staff. Within these groups are many subgroups, such as school board trustees, special education teachers, food service staff, team coaches, PTA reps, nurses, counselors, art teachers, music teachers, custodial staff, and YMCA, BGC, and parks and recreation staff. In targeting these groups, the toolkit is based on creating CATCH MVPs (i.e., high performers) amongst this group who lead, consistently produce results, and set a standard for success. A checklist and time lines are used as signposts to success.

So, how do I know so much about this partnership? Six years ago, I was brought on as a consultant to investigate the opportunity in introducing the CATCH program to Canada. FlagHouse has an office in Toronto, and we have the experiences and attributes that the management of the CATCH program at the University of Texas was looking for. My official title is CATCH Canada consultant, responsible for all CATCH program activity in Canada. I have been successful in building partnerships between federal and provincial levels of government as well as organizations such as the YMCA, Boys and Girls Clubs of Canada, community parks and recreation departments, and public health units. These partnerships were integral in providing the funding and credibility needed to launch the program in Canada and, more important, to sustain it. To date, in Canada more than 50,000 children have been affected by the program.

More important, you might ask, is why FlagHouse got involved in the partnership. What is in it for us? The CATCH program fit well with the strategies and goals of FlagHouse, such as offering programs, being community based, and providing goodwill to communities. At the time CATCH was the only school health program that had been proved to fight childhood obesity. It also represented an opportunity to promote the FlagHouse line of physical education equipment, so it seemed like a natural fit. Consequently, management approached me and asked whether I'd like to do some work on the partnership in Canada. In turn, the University of Texas and FlagHouse worked together, as partners on CATCH, to ascertain the resources necessary to fund my position. FlagHouse funded my position and tasked me to investigate the landscape in Canada, where I looked at the federal and provincial governments, nongovernmental organizations (NGOs), and essentially anyone who could help with this program. I then sought to make alliances with them. One example of success was a partnership with the YMCA in Canada, which played an important role in the launch of CATCH in Canada. I continue to promote the program in Canada and am involved in other marketing initiatives with FlagHouse Canada such as national contract development, and I have recently signed agreements with the YMCA of Canada to supply PE equipment to all of their associations across the country. This agreement was leveraged with the relationships made while developing the CATCH program in Canada. This is another example of the benefit of the program to FlagHouse, and it exposes the CATCH program to a wider national audience, a win–win for both groups.

The program continues to expand in both Canada and the United States. In 2012 the state of Texas launched 12 new grants through the Dell Foundation to reward youth. Also, Colin Powell presented to CATCH and gave kudos to the program. At this point, we've moved it to policy in the state of Texas, where our objective is to make CATCH part of the day-to-day effort against childhood obesity in the state.

Generally, for a partnership, I'd say we have four goals. First is to influence youth, to make a difference. Second is to be sustainable, so that our organization can continue to make progress and aid in the efforts against childhood obesity. Third, we seek to grow further from any successes that we have. Finally, CATCH, the partnership, has a mandate to grow internationally, including both to Canada and outside North America.

On the last issue, one that is highly relevant to partnerships and the protocol, one of our major challenges remains expanding the program beyond Texas, where it was born and where it is thriving. In principle, CATCH works. Lots of empirical research proves that it works, yet it remains a challenge in many jurisdictions outside Texas and Canada. In most cases, the big roadblock is politics. We hear about it all the time. Now, if you consider that it took us 20 years of ongoing efforts to establish ourselves in Texas, this may not be a surprise. Ten years ago, CATCH after school was originally run, for example, in Syracuse and Rochester (cities in New York State) with grants from the local hospital, but it has not grown at the same rate as it has in Texas. The role of FlagHouse also brings some challenges because some funders and governments have a bias against for-profits. My personal view is that this is wrong. Why should a great and successful program have borders? Look at the YMCA. They really got it and were willing to engage communities, and they have sustained and expanded the program.

You may also be interested to know why and how the CATCH–FlagHouse partnership has worked for so many years. I can think of a number of reasons, most of which align well with the protocol. First, the University of Texas CATCH team has always made the relationship with FlagHouse important, and they understand that the program can grow and flourish only with the support of a for-profit partner like FlagHouse. Second, internal champions are vital. When I think of the YMCA and its managers, their importance in the success of our programs when run there is immeasurable. It is about the teachers and instructors who want to make a difference in their communities, understand the unique qualities of the CATCH program, and promote them to their management. Third is not limiting the scope of your partnership and seeking other partners and programs. For CATCH and FlagHouse, we've also worked with the CDC, the Jared Foundation, the Boys and Girls Club, YMCA, MEND (Mind, Exercise, Nutrition, Do-It), Blue Cross, and many others. Fourth, the ability of the partnership to source resources from U.S. foundations and the Canadian government is key. These foundations are wonderful partners, and the program would not continue to exist if not for these partnerships. For example, our newest partnership is based in Texas with Baylor Health Sciences and the University of Texas and is funded in part by foundations and the Centers for Disease Control. The program, then, is vast and is based on a model of integrating the community, in which a child goes to a grocery store and can identify the CATCH characters in the produce section. Finally, I have learned through working in these types of partnerships that you do not have to be a large multinational organization to be involved in a successful partnership with an academic institution and that you can make a major difference at the community level.

FlagHouse is involved in a number of other difference-making community-based programs and represents the model of for-profit companies working with not-for-profit organizations for the greater good as well supporting a successful business model.

(continued) ▶

(continued) ▶

GLOBAL APPLICATION QUESTIONS

1. Check search engines and YouTube for CATCH. Review and learn about the intervention.

   a. Do you think it can work?

   b. What elements could make such a program a positive or a negative experience for the child?

2. List the benefits that FlagHouse receives from the partnership. In your opinion, is it worthwhile for FlagHouse, a small company? Take the example of a kit being provided to a new program with 2,500 participants.

3. Is FlagHouse taking advantage of the goodwill that it is generating through this partnership? If so, how are they doing that? If not, what would you recommend they do?

4. For public-sector partners beyond the University of Texas, such as other universities, how can FlagHouse persuade those partners to help them achieve their goals?

5. For the University of Texas and the CATCH program, how important or unimportant is it that they have a for-profit partner like FlagHouse? Explain.

6. The University of Texas' CATCH program has also partnered with the Jared Foundation (link to Subway). Is that a good idea? What alternatives might you have considered?

Partnership Examples

The purpose of this section is to illustrate, in a more concise manner than the University of Texas–CATCH–FlagHouse case study, partnerships between for-profit and not-for-profit organizations relevant to this book. There are hundreds more out there in the real world, and we encourage you to undertake a web search and have a look.

IBM Canada and Seven Ontario Universities

Recently, technology for-profit firm IBM, in particular its Canadian arm, announced a partnership with two governments and seven not-for-profit Canadian universities (all located in Ontario). The purpose of the partnership is to aid in a Canada-wide strategy to drive innovation and prosperity in the country by revamping how governments invest their dollars in research. The objective of the partnership is to create significant new capacity in supercomputing and cloud computing as a means to grapple with the huge amounts of data that researchers now work with in a variety of sectors.

IBM has agreed to contribute as much as CDN$175 million by 2014, in partnership with the government of Canada (CDN$20 million) and the government of Ontario (CDN$15 million). As universities face financial constraints, these kinds of projects with deep funding and a long-term commitment are very valuable. They represent a growing trend of governments seeking matching funds and more innovative and beneficial uses of their investments, particularly in research, R&D, and technology development. There is also the belief that these types of projects will have longer-term benefit for youth in terms of better jobs, a more competitive global economy, and opportunities for future generations. In addition to its financial investment, IBM will hire 125 new employees for its R&D center to coordinate and undertake work related to the projects with the seven partner universities—the University of Toronto, Western University, Queen's University, McMaster University, University of Waterloo, University of Ottawa, and University of Ontario Institute of Technology. A large data center will be built in Barrie. The initial focus of the partnership will be on research and development in areas such as neurological disorders, water conservation, and smart energy grids, reports say.

Examples of Public Private Partnerships

Table 10.2 outlines case examples related to partnerships.

Conclusion

Chapter 10 provides a case study and additional illustrations of the relevancy of *The Partnership Protocol* and partnerships in general to the physical activity, sport participation, and public health spheres. The CATCH case, in particular, informed by a key consultant on the project, provides validation for the protocol and its use by not-for-profit organizations.

TABLE 10.2 Key Learnings From Private Partnerships

Public-sector partner(s)	Private-sector partner(s)	Key learning	Reference
American Academy of Family Physicians	Coca-Cola	Partnership to develop consumer education materials. Importance of understanding potential conflicts of interests emphasized.	Marks and Thompson, 2011
PepsiCo and Kraft Foods	Save the Children	Collaborative effort to combat child malnutrition in Asia.	Kraak et al., 2009
Cadbury	UNICEF Canada	Money raised to support children and youth education in Africa through the sales of cobranded chocolate and candy.	Kraak et al., 2009
United States Department of Agriculture, National Center for Genome Research, Clemson University, HudsonAlpha Institute for Biotechnology, Indiana University, Washington State University	Mars Inc., IBM	Multiparty PPPs with more than one public-sector partner and more than one private-sector partner can be successful.	Genome Cocoa Project, www.cacaogenomedb.org
US AID, World Bank	Mars Inc., Waters Corporation	Partnered on the Global Food Safety Fund to address the challenge of food quality, both domestic and imported, around the world.	www.state.gov/r/pa/prs/ps/2011/11/177059.htm
Leyton Orient Community Sports Programme	Professional soccer teams	A partnership to introduce socially excluded groups to community activities through a yearlong sport program that included education, behavior modification, and rehabilitation focus to decrease drug use in the community.	Crabbe, 2000
President's Council on Physical Fitness and Sport, National Association of Sport and Physical Education; National Association for Sport and Physical Education	Kellogg Company	Kids in Action booklet helps make daily physical activity the foundation of a child's long and healthy life, based on the premise that children love to move, and provides advice to parents to play actively with their children.	Kids in Action, 2003

Public-sector partner(s)	Private-sector partner(s)	Key learning	Reference
Salt Lake City and the state of Utah, Salt Lake City Olympic Organizing Committee (SLOC)	Private investors	Description of the PPPs that led to the formation of the Olympic Games in Salt Lake City; discord between public and private interests resulted in doubtful economic viability of the facilities beyond the Games.	Andranovic, Burbank, and Heying, 2001
City of Sydney and Australian New South Wales government	International and Australian Olympic Committees	The Sydney Olympics, establishing a new model that the International Olympic Committee hoped would be adopted by other host countries to provide public accountability and include representation from all partners.	Wettenhall, 2003
World Swim Against Malaria	Largest net manufacturing company in Tanzania	Case study underlines the importance of trust, sacrifice, and championship as the three key themes of successful PPPs in developing countries.	Njaul, Mosha, and De Savigny, 2009
10 food and beverage companies	Various NGOs	Partnership to support various global programs of the International Food and Beverage Alliance (IFBA) to prevent non-communicable diseases and obesity.	Kraak et al., 2009
Coca-Cola	Red Cross	Partnership to support disaster response and preparedness for global humanitarian relief.	Kraak et al., 2009
Department of Energy, University of West Virginia	Multiple firms	Eastern Gas Shales Project illustrates ability of a government and a university to engage multiple private-sector partners.	www.washingtonpost.com/opinions/a-boom-in-shale-gas-credit-the-feds/2011/12/07/gIQAecFIzO_print.html
American Medical Association	Pfizer	Minority Scholar Awards, program targeted at underprivileged groups.	www.ama-assn.org/ama/pub/about-ama/ama-foundation/our-programs/medical-education/minority-scholars-award.page

CHAPTER 11

Challenges in Creating Effective Partnerships: Bias, Controversy, and Failure

Bringing together many minds, with many resources, for a common purpose fosters exciting promise for new physical activity and sport partnerships. Each contributor can add enthusiasm and creativity, but every new mind can also bring competing interests. Within partnerships, each organization ultimately is trying to further their own unique goals. This can create challenges in partnering, because the partnership needs to consider who holds the balance of power in decision making and dealing with outside competition, disconnect, and biases. Effective partnerships can overcome setbacks through well-developed planning that thinks through the partnership from everyday management and monitoring to responding to public feedback. The challenges are not minimal, but neither are they insurmountable in creating and maintaining effective partnerships that can make substantial contributions to increasing quality physical activity and sport participation and programming.

Excitement surrounds nascent partnerships. New teams are created; new ways of thinking come together; and new programs, products, and services can be launched. Along with embracing the initial enthusiasm, we need to consider how we will determine whether the partnership is successful and effective in reaching its goals. Partners, each with distinct goals and objectives, might have different perspectives on how to measure partnership effectiveness. To succeed, each partner's goals should be understood and measureable, and specific thinking and planning should be directed to what happens if, and when, things go wrong. Creating and sustaining effective partnerships includes many challenges; partners must achieve a delicate balancing of power in an environment of growing competition and public scrutiny. Having clear monitoring and responsiveness strategies in place and planning for setbacks can help partners minimize or avoid breakdowns and help organizations move forward beyond failure.

Measuring Partnership Effectiveness

Measuring effectiveness in partnerships can be viewed from two perspectives: effectiveness in outcome and effectiveness in process. In terms of the effectiveness in outcome, the partners may have different ways of measuring success. The private-sector partners often measure success in terms of return on investment, sales, revenue, and profits on a quarterly or annual basis, indicators that do not easily equate to successful sport and physical activity outcomes. In contrast, sport and physical activity effectiveness is often measured in the long term (e.g., higher fitness levels, decreased morbidity or mortality). With the multiple factors that contribute to overall fitness and other health indicators (e.g., nutrition, location, family composition, access to health care), isolating the role of a partnership on the health status of participants is difficult. For those reasons, many projects measure outcomes in terms of number of activities or events, number and diversity of participants, and proportion of repeat participators. Participation is measured because it is easy to measure, but health outcome is much more difficult to measure because it is long term and complex.

Effectiveness in process is well documented in the literature. In their study about successful private and public partnerships, Jacobson and Ok Choi (2008) listed nine factors that contribute to successful partnerships:

1. Specific plan or vision
2. Commitment
3. Open communication and trust
4. Willingness to compromise and collaborate
5. Respect and community outreach
6. Political support
7. Expert advice and review
8. Risk awareness
9. Clear roles and responsibilities

With a unified vision and mutually agreed-upon objectives and timetables, partnerships that engage in realistic, open, and honest communication are more willing to compromise, resolve challenges, and collaborate toward a building a successful partnership.

Trafford and Proctor (2006) recognized the need for good communication and openness in partnership planning while also reminding us that the direction and spirit or attitude of people in the community contribute to the success of a joint venture. In their COPED model, Trafford and Proctor (2006) developed a theoretical framework model for building comprehensive and productive relationships between public-sector organizations and private-sector companies. They recognized that the main challenge to effective partnering was establishing and maintaining strong communication between all levels of management; this meant overcoming barriers such as power imbalances, gender differences, physical surroundings, language, and cultural diversity. When priorities of the organization are unclear or underdeveloped, strategic planning processes (e.g., mission and objectives, environmental scanning, strategy formation, strategy implementation, and evaluation and control) could not be effective in delivering the anticipated outcome or process.

Elements of an Effective Partnership

The keys to effectiveness in creating strong partnerships in physical activity are good communication and planning between partners, and explicitly defined leadership roles and expectations of how the partnership will be monitored (see table 11.1). With adequate preparation, partners consider how the partnership could grow or change based on the response of participants and the community to be even more effective in delivering the partnership's promises.

TABLE 11.1 Elements of an Effective Partnership

Element	Key decisions
Clear communication and good planning	Who will communicate the partnership goals to the target group? How? What is the expected and desired outcome for each of the partners? How have short-term and long-term goals of each partner been considered in the planning? How will each partner's resources be used, and how will power be balanced? What social media tools will be used to communicate the partnership's messages?
Strong and defined leadership	Who will be responsible for leading and implementing the partnership initiatives in both the public and private spheres? Who will champion the partnership? Who will be responsible for ongoing partnership support?
Performance monitoring and responsiveness	How will the process effectiveness of the partnership be monitored? How will changes to the process be implemented if required? How will the partnership receive internal and external feedback? How will the outcome effectiveness be judged through both empirical and qualitative data?
Planning for setbacks	How will feedback change the process? How will disconnects be managed? How will setbacks be monitored and responded to by each partner? How will setbacks be communicated to the public and target audience? How can the partnership be terminated?
Future planning	How does the partnership fit with each partner's long-term strategies and ability or desire for future partnerships?

Clear Communication and Good Planning

The first element of an effective partnership is clear communication between partners from the onset. Each partner needs to lay out their expectations of the partnership objectives and progression. A carefully developed plan will substantially increase the probability of success of the partnership. Rosentraub and Swindell (2009) add that prenegotiations (specifically when dealing with a sport team) can be challenging but important. Planning will most often take the form of an extensive, detailed contract that clearly describes the responsibilities of both partners. In addition, timely and transparent mapping of all costs, revenues, and profitability aspects is a requirement for successful implementation (Sagalyn 2007). Partners should attempt to foresee areas of respective responsibilities and leadership, and good planning needs to include clearly defined methods of resolving conflict.

Strong and Defined Leadership

The second element of an effective partnership is strong leadership. In reviewing case studies of successful partnerships, Sagalyn (2007) found a common theme of skilled leaders and strong leadership. Weiermair et al. (2008) added that a successful partnership can result only if there is commitment from the top. The partnership can benefit when the most senior officials are actively involved in leading, supporting, or championing the programs or projects.

Performance Monitoring and Responsiveness

A third element of an effective partnership is monitoring during the partnership. Ongoing monitoring of the performance of the partnership can happen on a daily, weekly, monthly, or quarterly basis, based on the scope and goals of the partnership. In longer-term programs and projects, planning should consider how the partnership might change and evolve through its life cycle. According to Cousens et al. (2006), implementation and monitoring of evaluation policies, despite their importance, have largely been ignored in partnership planning. Babiak and Thibault (2009) furthered this sentiment by noting that public–private partnerships need observable and empirical performance measures to satisfy funding partners and government regulations. Monitoring and responding to public input (e.g., through social media tools discussed in chapter 3) can be an important measure of effectiveness and can help determine whether objectives have been satisfied.

Partnerships should have detailed specific targets and outcome indicators to analyze the benefits and costs of the partnership, as well as to consider the implications of any unexpected outcomes (Barr 2007). Van Kempen (2008) recommends that partners create a feedback loop that focuses on periodically assessing the strengths and weaknesses of the partnership by asking how well expectations were satisfied, how barriers could have been removed, and how outcomes could be improved. In the examination of Tennis Canada's aim to increase tennis interest in local communities, Vail (2007) noted that evaluating the partnership's success entailed measuring certain outcomes: number of new and maintained tennis participants, type and number of tennis programs, rallies and community partners, and the commitment of the program champion for an additional year.

In monitoring physical activity and health for Canadian youth, Active Healthy Kids Canada provides a report card grade based on how well certain initiatives and factors drive the quality and quantity of physical activity participation. Active Healthy Kids Canada (2009) highlighted the important (cognitive) role that physical activity plays in supporting and aiding student learning and performance outcomes (along with mental health, physical health, and body weight outcomes) as well as supporting the notion that youth with a disability and youth from low socioeconomic status backgrounds are at a disadvantage. Specifically, Active Healthy Kids Canada (2009, p. 3) notes the following:

> For example, a comprehensive Ontario school health initiative including physical activity as a key element indicated a 36 percent increase in reading and a 24 percent increase in math scores over a two-year period. A study of over 5,000 students by the U.S. Centers for Disease Control and Prevention indicated that girls with the highest levels of physical education participation had higher math and reading

scores. Another U.S. study of over 12,000 students indicated that daily physical activity was associated with higher math and reading achievement, echoed by an Alberta study of 5,000 students, which showed that active living had positive results on school performance. Healthy bodies and healthy minds are what Canada needs to have a strong, thriving society!

Active Healthy Kids Canada assigns specific grades in the report card and gives an overall assessment of an F for physical activity levels in Canada. This grade is based on evidence that most citizens in Canada are not reaching 90 minutes of daily physical activity daily despite the fact that physical activity levels have been increasing slightly (3 percent) since 2006. Still, only about 13 percent of Canadians take part in the recommended 90 minutes of exercise. The report card includes a number of component grades that assess factors related to physical activity, sport, and health. Notable components include Canadians' use of active transportation (biking or walking to school) at a D; screen time at an F (Canadian youth spend too much time in front of a screen); school physical education at a C−; and usage of facilities, programs, parks, and playgrounds at a D. External monitoring, like that of Active Healthy Kids Canada, can be important in targeting partnership goals in the broader scope of physical activity and health, and it allows the partners to respond to public realities.

Planning for Setbacks

Although every partnership strives to deliver effective programs and projects, successful partnerships also include planning for challenges and setbacks. The research of Babiak and Thibault (2009) points to the high rate of failure of partnerships, derived from factors including communication barriers, clashes in organizational visions and operating procedures, power imbalances, and the geographic locations of partners. Often these ineffective partnerships lacked ways to deal with the setbacks and did not have formal termination strategies in place. At the onset of building a partnership, partners need to consider the effects of failed partnerships. Frisby, Thibault, and Kikulis (2004) specify that these include public and employee discontent, loss of credibility and reputation, negative media exposure, and financial and resource losses.

To protect the public's investment and interests, Kennedy and Rosentraub (2000) suggest that contracts include provisions to specify damages or penalties that the private-sector partner will incur if the terms of the contract are not met. Some public–private partnerships include "clawback" clauses, which, as Kennedy and Rosentraub (2000) describe, "require the beneficiaries of public-sector incentives to repay a portion or all of the benefits they received if they fail to satisfy specific performance requirements" (p. 445). In partnering to create sport facilities, cities may attempt to negotiate a clawback that requires a professional sport franchise to repay certain amounts of community investment if the team leaves the city before a designated date. The penalties can diminish with time until the expiration of a lease, as per the negotiated contract.

In the examination of an arena built by a public–private partnership between the City of Toronto and the American Hockey League (AHL) Roadrunner team, Farag and Brittain (2008) noted that although game attendance was forecasted at 8,000, significant losses occurred when average attendance was much lower (approximately 1,200 fans). The public organization (City of Toronto) was spared losses because the partnership agreement allowed the city to reap the initial revenue first and required the private organization (the Roadrunner's team) to absorb the losses through a posted security deposit designed specifically for the case in which the partnership failed. The City of Toronto, without major losses in the Roadrunner partnership, was then able to move into a flat rental agreement with a second American Hockey League (AHL) franchise, the Toronto Marlies, which Farag and Brittain (2008) describe as more favorable for the city's return on investment.

Key Partnership Challenges

In her long career in public health, Dr. Becky Lankenau, director of the Centers for Disease Control and Prevention (CDC)–World Health Organization (WHO) Collaborating Center for Physical Activity and Health, has noticed that one of the challenges in the not-for-profit world is the existence of a culture that is counter to working with the private sector. Academic preparation usually doesn't include partnership building, so people often approach these collaborations with fear, mistrust, and lack of understanding of the potential benefits.

Numerous challenges stand in the way of the implementation of successful partnerships in sport and physical activity. First, we wrestle with the view that sport (and to some extent physical activity) is linked to professional sport and its rich athletes (as role models), rich owners, and vast resources. Second, the enormous attention paid to high-profile negative incidents in sport (e.g., abuse by coaches, doping, athlete misbehavior) affects people's view of sport and physical activity. Third, those outside physical activity and sport may not consider the association between sport participation and increased physical activity as important as causes like fighting cancer or promoting literacy or education. The reality is that many of the benefits achieved through sport and physical activity programs are realized in the long term (e.g., studies on health care show that the financial tax costs of inactivity are significant but not immediate). Finally, the public sector is assumed to be somewhat desperate. In this view, organizations take what they can get and are uncertain about the nature of their relationship with the private-sector partner, a mind-set that can undermine the effectiveness of the partnership.

Partners have to consider four challenges as they create, implement, and monitor their partnership: (a) how they will balance power, (b) how they will deal with competing interests and organizations, (c) how partnerships can work even when a seemingly large disconnect exists between the goals of the public and private organization, and (d) how they will resolve the inherent and perceived biases in their partnerships.

Balance of Power

There is an expectation that power should be balanced to create a mutually beneficial relationship. On the contrary, the benefits, power, and risks do not need to be balanced between partners, but partners do need clear expectations about their designated roles in the project. By assessing the capacity imbalance in a potential partnership, partners understand how each can offer support and where the other partner lacks resources or knowledge. As Babiak and Thibault (2009) explain, decision making and the coordination of work can sometimes be facilitated through the presence of a dominant partner. The level of asymmetry, which Babiak (2007) describes as the desire or ability to control another organization's operation or resources, needs to be agreed on by both partners. Although Vail (2007) indicated that a hierarchical relationship between collaborative partners can be a partnership challenge, Barr (2007) countered that hierarchy of authority in decision making is acceptable, and even desirable. As Babiak (2007) suggested, the power balance must be clearly articulated in building the partnership. There is a need to consider individual business and social compatibility, trust dynamics, and power relations rather than simply build on the assumption that partners are equals. Together, partners need to develop a vision of the partnership and then build effective images and systems to communicate, manage, and evaluate the partnership.

Competition

A partnership should be needs driven, and collaborative efforts must be aimed at meeting the needs of both partners. The culture and structures of the community must also be respected (UN 2007). But mutual respect and mutual trust do not always exist because there is a dichotomy of needs to attend to—those of the public partner and those of the private partner. A partnership can be competitive. As Babiak and Thibault (2009) explain, a primary concern for some sport organizations and not-for-profit agencies was that "although seemingly collaborating, many organizations involved in the (sport) system were competing on different levels of resources (money or other resources, such as athletes and coaches), legitimacy, or power" (p. 134). This situation manifests as tension between different levels of organizations (e.g., regional versus national interests or grassroots versus competitive interests). The actual needs and benefactors of the partnership need to be clear at the onset, as Joyner (2007) stated, to avoid ambiguity, resentment, confusion, and unrealized expectations. Without understanding each partner's ultimate aims, the partnership is compromised as partners move ahead independently, often in different directions.

The partners involved also need to consider how they will deal with competition from other organizations and how the competition influences the overall image of the partnership. Further investigation and consideration are needed into the competitiveness and disputes between public partners for private resources (e.g., recently the Vancouver Organizing Committee and

International Olympic Committee excluded the not-for-profit organization Right To Play from the 2010 Vancouver Olympics because there were conflicts among the group's private corporate sponsors, which has drawn much athlete and public criticism; see Starkman (2009)).

Competition also comes in the form of competing interests, space, and resources. Space for sporting activities is limited, and communities, organizations, and individuals may have different perspectives about what constitutes good use of space, which could result in competing interests trying to advance recreational sport, health, and environmental policies. Pitter (2009) described the conflict between an off-highway vehicle (ATV) group and active (human-powered) transportation (e.g., bike) supporters in the use of the trail systems in Nova Scotia, Canada. The creation of the Kieran Pathways Society, as Pitter (2009) described, championed with community allies to support the dedication of the trails for active transportation and healthy pursuits. Although the trails were developed in a government collaboration with the off-highway group, the active transportation network's differing beliefs about lifestyle and environment required them to work in partnership with the Nova Scotia government and local citizen groups to find a solution that best fit the community—a solution that could balance environmental, health, recreation, and political concerns.

Disconnect Between Partners and Goals

Partnerships are sometimes established even when disconnect appears to be present between the goals and values of the organizations involved. In some cases questions of ethics and integrity arise with the establishment of the partnership. Because sport sponsorship can be a significant tool for marketing, as Maher, Wilson, Signal, and Thomson (2006) describe, partnerships may arise in sport and physical activity that promote unhealthy products (e.g., high-fat or high-sugar products, tobacco, alcohol) that would seem to be counter to the goals and values of many sport and physical activity programs. Further, Maher, Wilson, Signal, and Thomson (2006) found that that sponsorship of sports popular with youth age 5 through 17 was heavily associated with unhealthy products, such as gambling, alcohol, and unhealthy foods. Disconnect between partners or goals may seem evident, such as the partnership between the Hershey Company, National Recreation and Park Association, USA Track & Field, and Athletics Canada in creating the Hershey's Track and Field Games. Is a disconnect present in a chocolate company's role in promoting the health of youth? An important point when considering the idea of disconnect in public–private partnerships in sport is a counterintuitive one; when considering the view of the private partner, the disconnect is often an asset that they are interested in (and are willing to pay a premium for). If the product being promoted (e.g., chocolate bars) is disconnected from the cause (e.g., obesity in kids), then the disconnect is of benefit to the private partner's objectives, as opposed to switching to a product (e.g., fruit bar) that is more connected to the cause.

Funding or Endorsement?
Challenge, Risk, and Bias

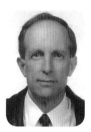

Art Salmon
Team Leader: Research, Ontario Ministry of Health Promotion

BIO

Art Salmon holds the position of team leader of research in the Sport and Recreation Branch of the Ontario Ministry of Health Promotion. He has primary responsibility for research and policy analysis in the area of physical activity and health. From 1991 to 2001 Art was national director of ParticipACTION. He then rejoined the Ontario government in the Ministry of Health Promotion. He currently is working with the World Health Organization and the U.S. Centers for Disease Control and Prevention in the design of national physical activity plans for Brazil, Chile, Russia, and Kuwait. He also is a member of the Canadian group that hosted the International Conference on Physical Activity and Obesity in Children in 2007 in Toronto.

GOVERNMENT AND HEALTH PROMOTION PERSPECTIVE ON PARTNERSHIPS

In November 1986 the first International Conference on Health Promotion, held in Ottawa, proclaimed the *Ottawa Charter for Health Promotion*. The charter includes this statement:

> The prerequisites and prospects for health cannot be ensured by the health sector alone. More importantly, health promotion demands coordinated action by all concerned: by governments, by health and other social and economic sectors, by nongovernmental and voluntary organization, by local authorities, by industry and by the media (World Health Organization, 2012).

Over the past 25 years numerous partnerships have been established between governments and nongovernment organizations, including business and industry, to enhance health and well-being.

FUNDING OR ENDORSEMENT?

As governments confront escalating budgetary deficits, in part a result of spiraling health care costs, they have found it increasingly attractive to seek the financial support and technical expertise of the private sector to assist in the funding and management of health promotion initiatives. In some quarters this arrangement is seen as the salvation for health promotion programs as tax-based budgets are reduced to address the deficit situation. Some have argued, however, that health promotion organizations, including governments, that accept funding from industries that manufacture and distribute unhealthy products are, in fact, becoming inadvertent pitchmen for those who are significantly contributing to unhealthy behaviors.

PUBLIC–PRIVATE PARTNERSHIPS: RISKS

Public–private partnerships in the field of health promotion are not without risk, and most governments are well aware that a cautious approach is both necessary and warranted. In examining public–private health partnerships involving the World Health Organization, Buse and Waxman (2001) characterized the WHO's involvement as a potential slippery slope. They noted that some critics position public–private partnerships with a discourse over the appropriate role of the state and public institutions in society. From the perspective of a national, provincial or state, or local government, an inadequately monitored partnership that lacks clear and concise terms of reference certainly has the potential to jeopardize the intended objectives of any project undertaken. As noted by Freedhoff and Hébert (2011) in an editorial focused on obesity and the food industry, "Health organizations, even when desperate for money or resources, should avoid co-branding with the food industry. At the very least, partnerships should comprise unconditional arm's-length grants with clauses limiting how corporations use health organization brands." A similar caution applies to governments, who, while willing to work with business and industry, would not want to be seen to be endorsing any particular private-sector brand or be associated with a product or service that is seen to be contributing to the health issue that is being addressed.

GLOBAL COMMITMENT TO HEALTH

At the sixth Global Conference on Health Promotion in Thailand, delegates ratified the *Bangkok Charter for Health Promotion in a Globalized World* (WHO, 2005). The charter identified actions, commitments, and pledges required to address the determinants of health in a globalized world through health promotion. The charter gave new direction to health promotion by calling for policy coherence, investment, and partnering across governments, international organizations, civil society, and the private sector to work toward four key commitments. These include ensuring that health promotion is central to the global development agenda, that health is a core responsibility of all governments and part of good corporate practice, and that it is a focus of community and civil society initiatives. The international health promotion community was sending a strong signal that progress toward a healthier world would require strong political action and broad participation by numerous sectors of society, including the private sector. In particular, recommendations from Bangkok identified the need for partnerships to (a) invest in sustainable policies, actions, and infrastructure to address the determinants of health; (b) build capacity for policy development, leadership, health promotion practice, knowledge transfer and research, and health literacy; and (c) partner and build alliances with public, private, nongovernment and international organizations, and civil society to create sustained actions.

(continued) ▶

(continued) ▶

CHALLENGE IN SHARING THE BURDEN OF HEALTH PROMOTION

At a time when the world is just beginning to emerge from the most devastating financial crisis since the Great Depression, governments are examining ways to reduce public-sector spending and fiscal deficits. Partnerships with the private sector may be seen as an effective mechanism to maintain programs and services by transferring the financial burden to business and industry. But as noted by Dixon, Sindall, and Banwell (2004), although such partnerships may have a stated aim of improving the health of the community, they may have been guided less by the ethos of the Ottawa charter and more by the interests of the various partners—namely, industry's need for credibility in making health claims and government's need to find preferred mechanisms for service delivery.

PROMOTING HEALTH: ASKING THE RIGHT QUESTIONS

Public–private partnerships have been seriously criticized in recent years. Buse and Waxman (Dixon et al. 2004) identified the types of issues that have arisen, such as the following: Are partnerships desirable, and under what circumstances, from a societal point of view? What are the appropriate criteria for the selection of candidate companies, industries, and activities, and how are such criteria developed? How can interactions be structured and monitored to avoid or deal with conflicts of interest? How can partnerships be made to function in accordance with principles of good governance? Governments at all levels must address these types of challenges and issues if they are to partner successfully with business and industry to advance health promotion activities.

GLOBAL APPLICATION QUESTIONS

1. Based on Salmon's perspective, what role can a government play in enhancing the effectiveness and responsible nature of partnerships between the private sector and the public sector in physical activity, sport participation, and public health?

2. Describe what Salmon means by "funding or endorsement."

3. Salmon's perspective clearly outlines the challenges, barriers, and risks that a government faces in considering participation in or support of partnerships. Based on his input, what role would you suggest that governments become involved in, if any?

Bias

When considering the ethics and integrity of partnerships, sponsorship agreements are considered. Rowe et al. (2009) questioned the scientific integrity of corporate-sponsored research, noting the need to disclose industry-sponsored research partnerships and financial interest in publications or presentations (interestingly, Rowe et al.'s research was sponsored by grants from Cadbury, Coca-Cola, ConAgra Foods Inc., General Mills, Kraft Foods, Mars Snackfoods,

PepsiCo, Procter & Gamble, Sara Lee, and Tate & Lyle). Other researchers echoed this concern. Boone (2004) noted the failure of some exercise physiologists to provide full disclosure of funding received from sport and nutritional supplement companies, yet "conflict-of-interest policies on the part of the investigators conducting sports supplement research have not been developed." To avoid any appearance of insincerity, each partner must ensure that its goals and objectives are understood by both the other partner and the public.

"For the food industry, partnership with health charities and health sector organizations are alluring. Doing so buys corporations credibility, ties brands to positive emotions attributed to their partnered organization and helps buy consumer loyalty—all good for the shareholders" (Freedhoff and Hébert, 2011).

Vocal opponents of public–private partnerships in health place specific criticism on the role that food companies play in shaping public health policy and skewing the public's perception on the causes of obesity (see Boone 2004; Butterworth 2011; Freedhoff and Hébert 2011; and Simon 2011). Part of the challenge is that when private food companies use public partnerships for clear economic gains, the partnership's ability to benefit the social good is suspect. Within funding food science and nutrition research, partnerships with the private sector are assumed to put scientific integrity at risk, but as Rowe et al. (2009) reported, there are ways to minimize the public- and private-sector conflict of interest to produce creditable research. Accordingly, Rowe et al. (2009) proposed eight principles to guide private sponsored research: (1) conduct or sponsor factual, transparent, and objective research that does not favor a certain outcome; (2) scientific investigators must remain in control of study design and research; (3) no remuneration should be geared to research outcomes; (4) written agreement should be in place for publication time frames; (5) financial interests in publications and presentations should be fully disclosed; (6) no undisclosed industry-sponsored paid authorship should be permitted; (7) guarantee appropriate auditor or reviewer access to all data and control of statistical analysis; and (8) require contract researchers to state their affiliations in research and publication. The guidelines that Rowe et al. (2009) proposed are not to discourage sponsored research but to halt the perceived (or real) bias and conflict of interest that can devalue the results.

With guidance from ParticipACTION's *Partnership Protocol*, it is possible to create partnerships between public and private partners (even big food or soda companies) that positively influence health and fitness and address obesity.

Avoiding Partnership Breakdown Through Good Management

Because partnering is challenging and often requires a long-term commitment, managing and building on the success of partnerships is more efficient than starting new, independent partnership processes. In this regard, van Kempen (2008) notes that building personal relationships and reporting about a program's success is important at the conclusion of a partnership to build potential for future partnering. Strong collaborative partnerships may draw new users to facilities for events, programs, and services and contribute to community development (Vail 2007). The spillover benefits of a successful partnership, which are largely intangible, could include increases in tourism, job creation, and general regional economic development (Rosentraub and Swindell 2009), which in turn can create conditions for new partnerships to deliver new sport events, programs, and products.

The literature points to the failure of many partnerships in effectively managing their collaboration; much time is spent in developing partnerships, but less time is devoted to creating specific plans of action, and even fewer hours are dedicated to the ongoing management of the partnership (Frisby, Thibault, and Kikulis 2004). Accordingly, Joyner (2007) noted that the fault of many public–private partnerships is that most of the time invested in the partnership is in the creation and negotiation phase rather than in managing the project. Further, partnering with private organizations may prove difficult for many community-based sport and physical activity organizations that are often volunteer driven and may have little or no financial management, reporting, and evaluation skills (Misener and Doherty 2009). Babiak and Thibault (2009) elaborated that the results of ineffective partnership management include project uncertainties, wasted time and effort, limited opportunity for success, and destruction of the partnership.

The importance of good management cannot be stressed enough. Even if partner management and leadership are unbalanced, partners must come to a consensus about each partner's role and accountability in managing the partnership (Cousens et al. 2006). Partners should aim to build predictable and long-term partnerships with processes that are well defined (UN 2007). To build effective partnerships, as Babiak and Thibault (2009) detailed, each of the partner's roles, responsibilities, and reporting channels must be coordinated and include clear direction about decision making, accountability, management, and evaluation.

Conclusion

From the time of partnership initiation, the project needs to be managed with clear definition, detailed planning and execution, and commitment to the project's close. Partners, both private and public, need to shed their unattainable expectations and not underestimate the scope and challenge that each partner undertakes in pursuing the partnership objectives. The challenges that organizations face in creating partnerships in physical activity and sport are difficult but not insurmountable. Considering competing interests from within and outside the organizations and understanding the perceived disconnect and biases that are inherent in the partnership can help partners move forward with effective partnerships. Overcoming the setbacks all comes down to clear and regular communication, good planning and management, strong and defined leadership (though not always equally balanced leadership), and preparation for overcoming future challenges. With proper monitoring and responsiveness, organizations can efficiently face challenges and maintain effective partnerships as they look to future opportunities.

The Science Behind Developing
The Partnership Protocol

In appendix B *The Partnership Protocol* is presented in its entirety to provide clear guidelines to organizations involved in public–private partnerships about how to undertake, implement, and manage partnerships in a responsible, effective, and risk-managed way. We, the authors of this book, were intimately involved in the process of developing *The Partnership Protocol*; one of us (O'Reilly) acted as the secretariat, and the other (Brunette) was a researcher. To validate these guidelines, we want to share the vast, stepwise research and consultation process that went into *The Partnership Protocol*.

The process that led to the building of *The Partnership Protocol* began with a conference call on August 7, 2009. The call was led by ParticipACTION, who invited a number of key stakeholders and experts to contribute their input in the area of partnerships between the private sector and the public sector in health, sport, and physical activity. During the call, participants sketched out a plan by which guidelines for responsible partnerships could be shared with industry and other stakeholders in 18 months. The plan included an extensive literature review, the creation of a representative steering committee, a detailed consultation process with key stakeholders, conference presentations, and a communicated and shared final document. Over the following weeks, a team was put together with representatives from the not-for-profit sector, the private sector, government, and academic communities. The committee was made up of the following members (with affiliations as of September 2009):

- Private-sector organizations
  - Mark Harrison, TrojanOne
  - Chris Lowry, Kellogg
  - David Moran, Coca-Cola

- Not-for-profit physical activity and sport organizations
  - Elio Antunes, ParticipACTION
  - Paul Melia, Canadian Centre for Ethics in Sport
  - Kelly Murumets, ParticipACTION (chair)

- Government
  - Art Salmon, Ontario Ministry of Health Promotion

- Research and academia
  - Peter Katmarzyk, Pennington Biomedical Research Center
  - Norm O'Reilly, Syracuse University (secretariat)
  - Mark Tremblay, University of Ottawa

The group, led by Murumets as chair and O'Reilly as secretariat, then undertook a multistep process to develop the guidelines in as diligent a way as possible and based on a limited budget.

The first step of the process was to review all previous research in the area of public–private partnerships and prepare a literature review on the topic. O'Reilly, at the time a faculty member at Syracuse University, led the effort, supported by Michelle Brunette of Laurentian University and Anne Warner of the University of Western Ontario. A nearly 200-page document was prepared in the fall of 2009 and shared with the steering committee for feedback. Following changes based on that feedback, the literature review was shared broadly during the consultation process with any interested party.

Building on the literature review, the steering committee drafted, redrafted, and altered many times the guidelines that eventually became *The Partnership Protocol*. Changes were made at various intervals internally by the authors and the steering committee and externally by using input from the consultation process, which included the following major steps, each of which was followed by a review of the feedback and changes to the draft guidelines.

- January 27, 2010—Murumets, as guest, and O'Reilly, as professor, ran a class and had MBA students complete a related case study on public–private partnerships (PPPs) at Stanford University's Graduate School of Business in a sport business class that O'Reilly was coteaching. The class of 55 students reviewed the draft and provided input.

- March 9, 2010—ParticipACTION, in collaboration with the steering committee, organized a full-day workshop of approximately 50 stakeholders in Toronto to share work to date, review a draft of the guidelines, and obtain feedback through organized work sessions.

- March 10, 2010—The steering committee followed the workshop with a second full-day session to address the concerns and findings of the workshop and build a more detailed draft of the guidelines. The session also included work on validating the guidelines with experts and planning for communication upon their completion.

- March 21, 2010—Murumets and O'Reilly presented the process and draft guidelines to a large session of approximately 100 attendees at the sixth annual Canadian Sponsorship Forum, held in conjunction with the 2010 Paralympic Games in Whistler, British Columbia. The session concluded with a voting session (using clicker technology) to obtain audience feedback on the work to date and an open Q&A session in which audience members could ask questions, provide feedback, suggest changes, or express concerns.

- May 7, 2010—Murumets, Tremblay, Katmarzyk, and O'Reilly presented the process and draft guidelines to a session of approximately 200 attendees at the International Conference on Physical Activity and Public Health (ICPAHP) held in Toronto, Ontario. The session concluded with a voting session (using clicker technology) to obtain audience feedback on the work to date and an open Q&A session whereby audience members could ask questions, provide feedback, suggest changes, or express concerns.

- June 2010—Global expert interviews. During the summer of 2010 O'Reilly conducted a series of expert interviews to review the draft guidelines. The expert interviewees were selected by the steering committee. Draft guidelines and the process to date were shared with interviewees before the interviews. Interviews typically lasted about 1 hour, although some took nearly 90 minutes. Following feedback from these experts, additional revisions were made. The experts interviewed included the following:

  - June 10, 2010—Dr. Derek Yach, senior vice-president, Global Health Policy, PepsiCo Global R&D, New York
  - June 11, 2010—Mr. Richard Pound, International Olympic Committee (IOC) member and partner, Stikeman Elliott, Montreal
  - June 15, 2010—Craig Larsen, executive director, Chronic Disease Prevention Alliance of Canada, Ottawa
  - June 17, 2010—Dr. Bruce Kidd, dean, faculty of Physical Education and Health, University of Toronto, Toronto
  - June 18, 2010—Bev Deeth, CEO, Concerned Children's Advertisers, Toronto
  - June 22, 2010—Stephen Samis, director, Health Policy at the Heart and Stroke Foundation of Canada (HSFC), Ottawa
  - June 23, 2010—Dr. Rhona Applebaum, VP and chief scientific and regulatory officer, Coca-Cola Company, Atlanta
  - June 24, 2010—Dr. Becky Lankenau, senior health scientist, National Center for Chronic Disease Prevention and Health Promotion, Atlanta

- August, September, and October 2010—Steering committee finalized guidelines. Decision made to present as *The Partnership Protocol*.

- November 2010—*The Partnership Protocol* is shared openly and at no charge.

The Partnership Protocol

The Partnership Protocol

Principles and Approach for Successful Private/Not-for-Profit
Partnerships in Physical Activity and Sport

October 2010

Dear Colleagues:

As the voice of physical activity and sport participation in Canada, ParticipACTION has had the opportunity to engage in a number of partnerships with private sector organizations for the advancement of our overall mission—a future in which Canadians are the most physically active on earth. Simultaneously, we have witnessed an increased need for partnerships between private companies and the sport and physical activity sector overall. Given the current scarcity of government resources and the potential benefits to both partners, it seems that partnerships are not only here to stay, but that they can advance our common interest: to increase the health and physical activity of a population that is increasingly at risk from its sedentary lifestyle.

In the summer of 2009, ParticipACTION assembled a group of leaders from several sectors to discuss the creation of guidelines for successful public-private partnerships. The aim was to assist not-for-profits in the fields of sport and physical activity to find, implement and sustain responsible, effective partnerships with the private sector, while simultaneously supporting individual missions and mandates.

This original group (comprised of representatives from academia, government, private corporations and not-for-profit organizations) completed a detailed literature review of public-private partnerships in the physical activity and sports world and created a Steering Committee to guide the process to develop the protocol itself.

Following completion of their background research and internal consultations, the Steering Committee launched a multi-stage consultation process. This included inviting input into four strategic partnership questions from fifty MBA students at the Stanford University Graduate School of Business and an invited group of thirty industry leaders and experts in Toronto. Their contributions served as the basis for a series of draft guidelines that were then presented to sixty-five delegates at the 2010 Canadian Sponsorship Forum in Whistler, B.C., for further feedback. Finally, the resulting guidelines were presented at the International Congress on Physical Activity and Public Health (ICPAPH) Conference in Toronto in May 2010.

The Partnership Protocol is a culmination of the advice of a broad cross-section of experts and interested parties who came together to offer their stories, experience and best practices to the community of not-for-profit organizations in the sport and physical activity sector. We hope you will find it useful in securing, building and strengthening positive partnerships that will enable your organization to continue to do its good work.

Sincerely,

Kelly D. Murumets
President and CEO, ParticipACTION
Chair of the Partnership Protocol Steering Committee

Overview:

The Partnership Protocol doesn't aim to answer the question of what is right for your organization, but rather to give you tools and information to help you find the best solutions possible for your needs.

Finding, developing and maintaining responsible and effective partnerships can be one of the most important aspects of work in the not-for-profit field. Successful partnerships can allow your organization to expand its programs, and broaden its audience and influence—in short, to do more of what you do, and to do it better. But partnerships can also present challenges. An unsuccessful partnership can jeopardize your organization, just as a successful one can advance it. So how do you make sure that the fit is right?

The Partnership Protocol is designed to help your organization answer that question, using the advice and best practices of a wide variety of experts from the world of academia, business and not-for-profit organizations. *The Partnership Protocol* focuses on three key areas of interest. Section 1, **Why Partnerships?** addresses the increasing need for not-for-profit organizations to enter into partnerships; Section 2 provides **Guiding Principles for Partnerships;** Section 3 suggests how to put those principles into practice in your organization's **Approach to Effective Partnerships.**

When considering these recommendations, it is important to remember that no two organizations have identical needs or concerns. Each organization is unique—in mission, leadership and aspirations—which means that each organization will have its own definitions for responsible and effective partnerships. *The Partnership Protocol* doesn't aim to answer the question of what is right for your organization, but rather to give you tools and information to help you find the best solutions possible for your needs. In the process, *The Partnership Protocol* provides an opportunity to debate, discuss and learn from other groups' partnerships. The ultimate goal of *The Partnership Protocol i*s to increase capacity in the physical activity and sport sector.

1. Why Partnerships?

NFPs are increasingly exploring and entering private sector partnerships as a means to generate additional resources and to provide for the long-term viability of the sector overall. An effective partnership requires both partners to have a vested interest in the partnership and to agree to work together in the best interests of the partnership.

The challenges facing not-for-profit (NFP) organizations that focus on physical activity are at an all-time high. Resources are few and the need is high. But from these increasing challenges come increasing opportunities. NFPs are increasingly exploring and entering private sector partnerships as a means to generate additional resources and to provide for the long-term viability of the sector overall.

Mutually Beneficial Outcomes for Partners

Sharing resources can allow both partners to achieve their individual goals. Mutual benefits may include enhanced value for investment in achieving objectives; sharing human resources, assets and expertise; improvements in productivity; improved distribution of products/programs and ideas; reduced risk or shared risk; and growth[1].

The Growing Physical Inactivity Crisis

Physical fitness levels of youth aged 6 to 19 years, both male and female, have been declining dramatically for three decades.[2] Similarly, fitness levels of adults aged 20-69 years have also declined.[3] Sport participation rates in Canadian youth aged 15-18 declined from 77% to 59% between 1992 and 2005 and declined in Canadian adults from 45% to 28% during the same period.[4] Physical inactivity leads to a host of chronic degenerative conditions and premature death.[5] The economic burden of physical inactivity in Canada is estimated at $5.3 billion annually and the annual burden to the healthcare system is estimated at $2.1 billion.[5] Regular physical activity, including sport participation, is associated with as much as a 30% reduction in all-cause mortality rates[6].

Scarcity of Government Resources

In many countries, government support to NFP organizations is dwindling. This decrease in support has generally stemmed from cutbacks in government spending on physical activity and sport, and/or an increase in the proportion of tax dollars required for core health care and education services.[6] Governments also expect the organizations that they do support to generate additional funding from other partners.

Escalating Competition for Resources

As Western society begins to recognize the severity of the physical inactivity crisis, more organizations are being formed to deal with specific and important causes. In addition, some NFPs are using increasingly sophisticated strategies and technological tools[7] for getting the attention of government funders. This has created a competitive environment in which NFP organizations vie for limited government dollars.

As a result of these factors, NFPs are increasingly considering partnerships with the private sector. At the same time, the private sector is increasingly interested in the business and branding opportunities offered by NFP physical activity and sport organizations. While there are many motivating factors that establish such partnerships, developing and activating these partnerships raises both philosophical and practical questions.

Given the current government funding climate and the potential benefits of positive partnerships with the private sector—and with the strong agreement of our consulted experts—we have concluded that partnerships are essential to advancing the aims of the physical activity and sport sector, and to working toward our shared goal of a healthier, more physically active society.

What is an Effective Partnership?

When discussing partnerships, it is important to first reach a shared definition. A NFP/private sector partnership is a strategic alliance between two parties in which one partner is a not-for-profit physical activity or sport organization and one partner is a for-profit corporate organization which operates independently of government and has a goal for the partnership of providing a positive return to shareholders.

The Partnership Protocol bases its understanding of *effective* partnership on key underlying views of partnership in the physical activity and sport context.

An effective partnership requires both partners to have a vested interest in the partnership and to agree to work together in the best interests of the partnership.

Partnerships should be conceptualized as on a continuum. The position on the continuum depends on the strength of the partnership (i.e., commitment and longevity of the partnership) and level of influence on the other partner's goals, objectives and actions.

At one end of the continuum, we find the most effective partnerships—strong, mutually beneficial partnerships, often grown from an initial sponsorship in which both organizations are mutually supportive and contributing to the partnership equally. In the physical activity and sport sector, these ideal partnerships typically involve pooled financial, product and human resources to create facilities, events, products and programs.

At the other end, there are weaker partnerships. These partnerships are typically donations or grants made to an NFP by an individual or an organization with little ask and engagement from the private sector organization in the NFP and its work.[1]

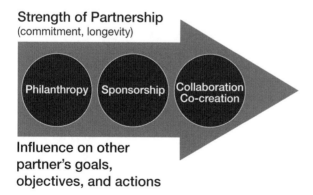

Strength of Partnership
(commitment, longevity)

Philanthropy   Sponsorship   Collaboration Co-creation

Influence on other partner's goals, objectives, and actions

2. Guiding Principles for Partnerships

The success of your partnership is dependent on shared goals and vision and an understanding of how the partnership will unfold through each stage of your joint project.

In order to support NFPs in the sport and physical activity field to find, establish and grow effective and responsible partnerships with the private sector, *The Partnership Protocol* endorses the following Guiding Principles.

Share Each Other's Equity

Share and value the assets that each partner brings to the table. An effective partnership will leverage and extend each partner's assets, so that the partnership's scope is greater than either organization's individual potential. Ensure that the partnership will further your own mission, but will also offer a return on investment for your partner organization and will contribute to the overall societal goal (e.g. increased awareness and/or behaviour change in physical activity and sport participation).

Stay True to Who You Are

Your equity and your brand are your organization's most important assets and cannot be sacrificed for attractive amenities in a partnership. Seek a partner who will be able to offer an equity that is equal to your organization's equity. A partner should be able to help you establish credibility and garner incremental recognition. The corporate "match" must be compatible with your values, goals and branding. Safeguard your organization's credibility and reputation: stay true to who you are.

Acknowledge and Manage Risk

Consider the risks and rewards of each potential partner and understand the implications of working with that organization. Is the reward of the partnership's possibilities equal to, or less than, the risks to your NFP organization?

If you acknowledge upfront any real or perceived disconnects between your cause and your potential private sector partner, you will be able to plan for possible problems and consider how you will deal with them in order to maintain the integrity of your projects. Remember that many businesses are interested in making a more positive societal impact, and working with credible NFP organizations can help companies to achieve these altruistic goals, as well as their business objectives.

Create Compelling Communications

An effective partnership needs to be built on a legitimate and relevant platform. A successful partnership ensures that all stakeholders hear this story and both parties share the societal recognition.

Be a storyteller before, during and—most importantly—after the partnership. This will increase the learning for the partners and for others, informing future partnerships and helping to address potential criticism and negative or inaccurate perceptions. Your storytelling must show how the partnership supports the public interest. If you cannot articulate the societal benefit of the partnership, seriously consider whether the partnership is viable.

Be sure that both partners take an active role in communicating the partnership to government, so that governments continue to recognize their role in addressing the societal need for increased physical activity. By creating successful campaigns and compelling communications, you and your partner organization can help entice the public sector to join the cause or continue its support.

Inspire, Motivate and Activate Your Stakeholders

Talk to all the parties that the partnership touches—government, bloggers, media, consumers, donors, volunteers, members, supporters and advocates—to further the understanding of the partnership and to generate excitement about the possibilities it creates. Remember that those parties are not merely entities, but are made up of real people. Cultivate relationships with key individuals in each of these areas. Make each of these people understand that they have a definite role in the partnership's success and the societal benefit it creates. Stakeholder engagement should be sought at each stage of the partnership, from design and implementation, right through to your final evaluation.

Be Clear

The success of your partnership is dependent on shared goals and vision and an understanding of how the partnership will unfold through each stage of your joint project. You and your partner must clearly define success, measurable objectives, expectations and roles. Ensure that a process is in place for clear, regular communication, coordination, accountability, reporting, approvals and conflict resolution. It is also important to recognize how external factors may impact the individual partners and their shared projects (e.g. recession, Olympics). Ensure that the partnership builds and maintains the elements of any good personal or business relationship: honesty, trust, respect and transparency.

Measure and Evaluate

Good measurement is essential to good partnerships. Evaluate your partnership from initiation and on through major milestones, to assess whether the association is having a positive impact—on your organization, your partner's business, and society. Use reliable and accurate evaluation techniques, metrics and interpretations to continue to identify what is working, realize opportunities for improvements and determine a suitable course of action for the future.

3. Approach to Effective Partnerships

Be flexible to the needs of your partner and communicate often and openly—informally and at established check-in points.

The Partnership Protocol has identified the following steps, strategies and recommendations to help your organization facilitate responsible, effective and enduring partnerships with the private sector.

The Approach is organized into three phases: **Assessing, Building** and **Managing the partnership.**

Phase 1: Assessing Potential Partners

Choosing the right private sector organization to partner with can make all the difference to your NFP organization, affecting the success of your projects, your organization's brand and your ability to fulfill your mandate. Here are some things to consider when making your choice:

1) Do the organizations share a common interest or a shared goal in advancing sport and physical activity? Your potential partner should have an understanding of the measures of success for both partners, the desired social health and wellness benefits of the partnership and the process to achieve outcomes.

2) Develop a profile of the potential partner and review internally. Does this private sector partner offer opportunities for a successful, long-term partnership?

3) Identify the expertise, resources, reach and assets that the prospective partner would bring to your partnership and to your organization. Assess the partnership opportunity by considering what else might be accomplished with the time and resources your organization will invest in the partnership.

4) Identify or validate champions for the prospective partnership—one at your NFP and one at the partner organization. These people can ensure ongoing high level dialogue and commitment to the partnership's objectives.

5) Review your potential partner's target audiences, considering points of crossover with your organization's audiences— current and desired. How might this partner help you broaden your organization's communication to new audiences or improve your reach into current audiences?

6) Evaluate the relative risks and rewards and understand the implications of working with potential partners. Can the value of the partnership be communicated and defended?

7) Consider the overall brand of your potential partner and its current partner mix. How will your partnership fit?

8) Assess both parties' capacity to fulfill partnership promises. Do you both have the will and the means to deliver? Is there shared accountability and responsibility to partnership outcomes?

9) Consider how the partnership will align with your organization's values, brands and cultures. If you identify disconnects, consider how these might be balanced. Note that some potentially controversial companies are interested in partnering with the sport and physical activity sector in order to offset the disconnects between their reputation and our sector's positive

public image. Are there ways to build the partnership so that these disconnects work to the advantage of your NFP, such as making sure that the company's contribution represents a fair and equitable value for the risk? Could this partnership prevent other partnerships or harm your organization's potential activities in the future? If the controversy is unwarranted, consider how best to overcome opposing viewpoints and be prepared to defend these viewpoints in the public domain when challenged.

Phase 2: Building Partnerships

Building a partnership involves discovering suitable evaluation metrics and solidifying the relationship with an agreement. This stage lays the groundwork for building an effective, enduring and fair partnership that will allow both partners to pursue their objectives.

THE RELATIONSHIP

The nature of the relationship between an NFP and its private sector partner is fluid, and real conflicts and problems can easily arise. But there are things your NFP organization can do to help mitigate these potential difficulties:

1) Work to achieve internal support for the partnership in both organizations, working at the levels of the board/ ownership, management and staff, but note that even in a signed partnership agreement, it is unlikely that any partner will have 100% support.

2) Work with your partner organization to determine the controllable elements of your partnership and its projects, and decide how these will be managed and communicated, internally and to your stakeholders and the public.

3) Establish clarity in the partnership by developing and achieving collaborative agreement on the shared vision, goal(s) definition of success, expectations, rules of engagement, and measurable objectives.

4) Understand that individual relationships are as important as organizational ones. Encourage members of your NFP to take time to develop these relationships with their counterparts in the private sector organization.

5) Be flexible to the needs of your partner and communicate often and openly—informally and at established check-in points.

6) When conflicts arise or when your organization's interests and those of your partner diverge, be clear and upfront about the nature of the disagreement.

7) Manage the relationship in a way that the public will understand and communicate it effectively to your wider audience. This management might include the creation of a crisis management plan to handle any possible large-scale objections to the partnership. This plan would outline key messages and Q&As, and specify (and educate) a potential spokesperson to counter negative perceptions, internally or externally.

8) When dealing with a private sector corporation, consider the use of a "less risky" brand within their corporate family or the corporate brand as the label for the partnership. Consider both product brands and the overall corporate brand that reflects the partnership. However, as stated earlier, you must ensure that the partnership builds and maintains honesty, trust, respect and transparency. To that end, the partnership must never hide or deny the identity of the corporate parent.

9) Establish a process of accountability and follow it, delivering as promised.

10) Remain mindful of the culture of each partner and work to respect them.

11) Be honest and transparent with your private sector partner in all aspects of the partnership.

12) Remember that long-term partnerships are more desirable than short-term sponsorships or partnerships. Build the partnership in a positive manner, with a view to extending any successful project or re-engaging your partner for future collaborations.

THE AGREEMENT

Partnership agreements can take many forms. The length of the document should reflect the nature of the relationship and the scope of the partnership. The agreement needs to be comprehensive, drafted by the people who will implement it, reflect the partners' relationship and be reviewed and approved by legal experts—preferably by lawyers who specialize in sponsorships.

Regardless of length or style, all partnership agreements should be ethical, purposeful, thorough, principled, transparent, legally viable and enforceable.

When drawing up the partnership agreement, your NFP should also consider:

1) Clearly outline each partner's role, responsibilities and deliverables. This should include the internal, as well as the external, roles of each partner.

2) Clearly outline the granting of rights (e.g. use of logo or trademark), copyrights, confidentiality, ownership of products developed (including product life after partnership).

3) Note in detail jurisdiction, termination/ exit clauses, definitions (what is "contract", who is "partner", what is "category", etc.) and related terminology, dispute resolution plan (e.g. third party), force majeure and signing authority.

4) Lay out responsibilities for insurance, liability, resources contributed (cash and/ or in kind), communications commitments, controls on the post-contract behaviour of both parties and exclusivity.

5) Ensure that the resources to be invested by the private sector partner will allow the partner to meet both your partnership's objectives and their own business objectives.

6) Articulate the amount of resources that both partners will allocate towards the fulfillment of the partnership, resulting in a turnkey approach to the partnership.

7) Develop a Legacy Plan and decide what enduring benefits will remain for both partners, after the partnership concludes.

8) Detail the plan, resources and timing for evaluation.

9) Solidify a clear process to approve changes to the agreement.

Phase 3: Managing the Partnership

The goal of the Partnership Management phase is to ensure that the partnership 'lives' as it was planned in the agreement and is communicated effectively to all stakeholders.

PROJECT MANAGEMENT

It is imperative to reach an agreement about the vision, goals and measurements of success for your partnered project. Participants in this agreement should include the project team, your NFP's management and your partner's representatives on the project. To ensure that the plan stays on track, you will need continuous and effective communication between both parties and all the individuals involved from the two organizations, along with a controlled scope of activity. Management at both partner organizations must be verbally and practically supportive of the project and the staff carrying out the project. Designating a senior champion for the project from both organizations sets the tone and helps showcase the partnered project as a priority for the organizations.

Key steps for an effective project management in an NFP/private sector partnership include:

1) Project Initiation:

   • Agree at the outset, and include in the Agreement, the shared vision, goal(s), intended outcome and success criteria.

   • Articulate clearly project ownership, accountability and decision-making processes.

   • Approve partnership agreement.

2) Project Definition:

   • Engage all relevant internal and

external stakeholders in initial consultation and incorporate their feedback and previous lessons learned.

- Confirm concept and budget.

- Identify project team from within both partner organizations, ensuring representation from all departments critical to the project's success.

- Agree on project objectives and how objectives will be measured and reported.

3) Project Planning:

- Develop and approve a detailed Work Breakdown Structure that defines key milestones and deliverables

- Develop an activity plan that outlines key activities, responsibilities and timelines for both partners. Depending on the project, the activity plan should include plans for content development, creative development, production and fulfillment, a website, internal and external communications and risk management (including planning for a potential negative response from media), evaluation, financial management, reporting and approvals. Include a Gantt chart to make it easy to follow progress and detailed budget.

- Establish regular project team meetings, both for the core team for ongoing project implementation, monitoring and co-ordination; and for the senior team members to ensure enduring strategic alignment to the vision, goals and direction of the project.

4) Project Execution:

- Implement the project according to the plan, with regular status updates and adjustments to the plan as needed.

- Monitor progress regularly by reporting agreed metrics against objectives to determine if project is on track or if course correction is needed.

- Monitor budget against actual expenditures regularly and adjust forecasts as needed to ensure project is delivered within budget.

5) Project Close:

- Complete evaluation and project reporting.

- Debrief with project team to identify successes, challenges and lessons learned.

- Implement strategy to renew agreement, if appropriate, or execute a smooth and respectful exit strategy, should either party decide to terminate the relationship.

- Create an exemplary ending. Ensure that the partnership is completed in a positive and respectful manner, laying the groundwork for both partners to create future relationships between other parties in the NFP and private sectors.

EVALUATION

Evaluation of the project must occur from three separate perspectives: 1) the perspective of your NFP organization; 2) the perspective of the private sector partner, and 3) the sport and physical activity cause itself. Within each of these evaluations, a measurement must be taken both of the outcomes of the project and of the processes followed.

Evaluation is not simply a tool to employ at the end of a project. To create an effective final evaluation, baseline measures should be taken or established before the partnership is even launched and appropriate metrics should be adopted for the active partnership and for the post-partnership measurement. The evaluation can be carried out internally by each partner, or by an external third party, according to the project agreement.

1) What to Measure:

Intended/Unintended Benefits and Consequences: Gauge these benefits and consequences through the lens of both partners achieving their objectives as well as the partnership's impact on society though behaviour change or increased awareness.

Contract Fulfillment: Were all stated deliverables achieved?

Success of Project (Business): Note achievement of business objectives for each partner, externally (sales, reach, brand effects, credibility, reputation, awareness, impressions, return-on-investment, corporate responsibility) and internally (employee engagement, employee satisfaction with partnership, impact on employee turnover).

Success of Project (Societal): Gauge partnership's impact on health and wellness cause (what results can be seen in behaviour change and/or awareness?).

Partner Satisfaction: Measure the following types of factors:
- Overall Satisfaction (i.e. trust, respect, quality of collaboration, budget, etc.).

- Adherence to Planned Investments (Did either partner invest more resources than planned for in the agreement?).

- Impact of United Efforts (Did the partnership allow the parties to accomplish something they could not have achieved on their own?).

- Willingness to Continue Partnership (through renewal or expansion).

2) How to Measure:

Be transparent and comprehensive in the methods you are using to measure the partnership. Incorporate:

- Quantitative measurement (e.g. surveys, comparisons to similar situations/industries)

- Empirical measurement

- Qualitative measurement (e.g. interviews and testimonials)

Plan for longitudinal studies, establishing benchmarks, using repeatable methods, etc.

Use 360° Analysis: Obtain evaluations from third-party stakeholders (e.g. expert interviews,

value assessments), the sector and the public (e.g. community surveys) including at the grassroots level.

Undertake independent third-party partnership evaluation to:

- Determine if partnership has impacted ability of either partner to attract new partners

- Conduct opportunity cost analysis for partnership

COMMUNICATING THE PARTNERSHIP
The final stage of the Approach to Effective Partnerships is communicating the outcomes of the NFP/private sector partnerships—telling the story of the partnership and its benefits to both internal and external audiences.

Internal Storytelling: Stories from past and current partnerships should be communicated widely within your organization. This storytelling helps your organization to avoid past failures, learn from past challenges and build on past successes. This storytelling can be achieved through blogs, articles in newsletters, presentations at meetings and conferences, postings in staffrooms, website reports, etc.

External storytelling: Partners should jointly communicate their successful experiences ("best practices") and unsuccessful experiences ("learnings") to other NFPs and private sector organizations, with an aim to improve sector-wide understanding of partnerships, benefitting the shared cause of sport and physical activity. Methods to communicate these stories include industry publications and websites, scientific journals, professional society websites, direct mail or e-mail, trade reports and conferences.

Corporate partners will also want to tell a story about the positive societal impact they achieved through their NFP partnership (within their own industry and to their customers and stakeholders). It is essential that these communications include objective, independent data that clearly indicates how both parties contributed to the partnership's success. Ensure that your NFP organization's role in the partnership is effectively presented in their stories.

Moving Forward Together: Putting *The Partnership Protocol* to Work

This document is designed to help your NFP organization to find, implement and sustain responsible, effective partnerships with the private sector while supporting your mission and mandate. It is also a record of an ongoing dialogue of combined resources, counsel and best practices. This dialogue will be strengthened by further input—from experts, from the sport and activity sector, and also from NFPs with other mandates. The more NFPs use and discuss these issues, the more we strengthen our ability to create good partnerships with the private sector, so that we can effect positive change in the society we share. Here are a few ways you can continue the conversation:

- Share with your board, staff and colleagues

- Consider sharing it with your current partners

- Audit your existing partnerships against the guidelines, score how you are doing and identify things to change when you renew

- Discuss with your own social networks and share ideas

- Use when assessing and establishing new partners

- Use this document as a template for other sectors (e.g. nutrition, health)

- Ask questions. Use *The Partnership Protocol* as a template that you can customize to suit the needs of your organization, adding and changing it based on your own experience.

- Learn, challenge and share this and other resources and your evolving best practices with others in the sport and activity sector and with NFPs with other mandates. Continue the dialogue.

Contact Information:

ParticipACTION
2 Bloor Street E.
Suite 1804
Toronto, ON, M4W 1A8
416-913-1511
info@participACTION.com
www.participACTION.com

Acknowledgements

The Partnership Protocol, Principles and Approach for Successful Private/Not-for-Profit Partnerships in Physical Activity and Sport was developed with the expertise, insight and best practices shared by a diverse set of over 300 stakeholders. A sincere thank you also to the project's Steering Committee for their vision, guidance and expertise throughout the process. Steering Committee members included:

- Elio Antunes, COO and VP of Partnerships, ParticipACTION

- Mark Harrison, President, TrojanOne

- Dr. Peter Katzmarzyk, Associate Executive Director for Population Science, Pennington Biomedical Research Center

- Chris Lowry, Vice President, Nutrition & Corporate Affairs, Kellogg

- Paul Melia, President and CEO, Canadian Centre for Ethics in Sport

- David Moran, Director, Public Affairs and Communications, Coca-Cola Canada

- Kelly Murumets, President and CEO, ParticipACTION

- Dr. Norm O'Reilly, Associate Professor of Sport Business , University of Ottawa

- Dr. Art Salmon, Team Leader, Ministry of Health Promotion, Government of Ontario

- Dr. Mark Tremblay, Director, Healthy Active Living and Obesity Research, Children's Hospital of Eastern Ontario Research Institute

End Notes:

1   O'Reilly, Norm (2010), "Public-Private Partnerships in the Sport and Physical Activity Contexts", a literature review completed as a pre-curser to this project. Available upon request from ParticipACTION.

2   Tremblay, M.S., Shields, M., Laviolette, M., Craig, C.L., Janssen, I., & Connor Gorber, S. (2010). Fitness of Canadian children and youth: Results from the 2007-2009 Canadian Health Measures Survey. *Health Reports*, 21(1):7-20.

3   Shields, M., Tremblay, M.S., Laviolette, M., Craig, C.L., Janssen, I. & Connor Gorber, S. (2010). Fitness of Canadian adults: Results from the 2007-2009 Canadian Health Measures Survey. *Health Reports* 21(1):21-36.

4   Sport participation in Canada, 2005. *Culture, Tourism and the Centre for Education Statistics.* Vol. Catalogue no. 81-595-MIE – No. 060: Statistics Canada XPE, Health Reports, Vol. 21, no. 1, March 2010.

5   Katzmarzyk PT, Janssen I. (2004).The economic costs associated with physical inactivity and obesity in Canada: an update. *Can J Appl Physiol.* 29 (1):90-115.

6   Andersen, L.B., Schnchr, P., Schroll, M., et.al. (2000). All-cause mortality associated with physical activity during leisure time, work, sports and cycling to work. *Arch Intern Med.* 160: 1621-1628.

EPILOGUE

After many pages, examples, illustrations, and research, has this book accomplished anything? Does the presentation of *The Partnership Protocol* help not-for-profits in this world? Is the informed input of more than a dozen experts on various elements of partnerships useful?

We, the authors would argue a resounding yes!

OK, we agree, we're biased, but let us summarize. Consider these half-dozen key points or ideas.

First, controversy exists here, but public–private partnerships aren't as negative as they are often portrayed. There is no question that if not undertaken and managed in a reasonable way, certain partnerships can cause impacts on the general population that are counter to the goals of the public-sector partner. For example, a corporation who has products and brands that are unhealthy will benefit in terms of image, brand, and eventually sales of those products and brands from strategically associating with a not-for-profit whose images are positive. That's that. But this book argues (convincingly, we'd say!) that a private-sector organization can achieve those goals in many ways. Marketing, after all, is vast and effective! So, a private-sector organization has options about where to invest their resources. Why shouldn't we convince them to invest those resources in physical activity, sport participation, and public health?

Second—and this is an important underlying premise of this book—is that the leadership of not-for-profit organizations can choose whether or not they want to consider partnerships with the private sector. Even if a board of directors or senior management team decides to pursue a partnership, the reality is that many not-for-profits do not have much to offer a private-sector partner from a marketing perspective (remember, philanthropy is not the focus of this book). But regardless of private-sector interest, a not-for-profit must first decide whether a partnership is something that they even want to consider. Some boards and managers have opted not to consider this route. There is no problem with that, none at all! The choice is theirs. This book is not for them. It is for those who do decide to go down this route. For those who do, we believe that the elements of this book, particularly *The Partnership Protocol*, provide the strategic and tactical direction to build, manage, and evaluate partnerships with the private sector in a responsible way, in which the benefits to the not-for-profit and its cause far outweigh any negative outcomes, which can be mitigated to a significant extent, if not eliminated. Careful consideration of the protocol and the various strategic elements provided in the book (e.g., champions, corporate social responsibility, role models, sponsorship, fund-raising) will provide not-for-profits in physical activity, sport participation, and public health with the ability to generate new resources for their programs and activities and manage the associated risks in a responsible way that protects their organization, brand, and membership.

Third, a partnership with the private sector needs to be viewed by a not-for-profit organization as an option, an alternative amongst many that they can consider in the context of constrained resources (i.e., increased competition among more and varied not-for-profits for increasingly limited government and foundation funding). In many cases, not-for-profit organizations in physical activity, sport participation, and public health rely heavily on government funds and foundation support. Because this support may be cut or offered to a competing not-for-profit organization (common in the current climate), pursuit of new resources has become a top priority for many boards and managers.

Fourth, disconnect, disconnect, disconnect. If your not-for-profit organization has decided to embark on partnerships with the private sector and if such partners are interested in your organization and your cause, the disconnect is a vital concept to understand. As described in detail in the book, the disconnect (i.e., the difference in images between the cause and the products or brand of the private-sector partner) is, from a marketing perspective, not a bad thing. Indeed, in many cases the disconnect is the source of the private sector's interest in a partnership with you, and it is valuable to you when negotiating how much the partnership will generate for your organization. Yes, a disconnect is a premium.

Fifth, embarking on a partnership with the private sector is described as a major undertaking, a proposition with risk, and a process requiring diligent project management and smart evaluation. If your not-for-profit organization decides to go this route, this book provides a variety of strategies, tools, and recommendations to be successful and responsible. Indeed, *The Partnership Protocol* outlines a clear, stepwise approach to achieving a successful partnership. Make this a priority. Allocate human resources to manage and build a strong relationship with your private-sector partner. Engage champions. Collaboratively build fund-raising events and activities. Service the corporate social responsibility needs of your private-sector partner.

Finally, we would like to emphasize, as *The Partnership Protocol* does, the importance of "storytelling" in partnerships. Share successes and opportunities with your boards, your staff, your membership, your participants, your fans, and your donors. Develop a media plan to share externally. Sure, some media is expensive, but your website, an e-blast, a blog, and a social media post are not resource intensive and will produce some impact. Indeed, if the story is particularly good and a tad controversial (as these partnerships often are), it may get more coverage than expected. Do not be afraid of this—manage it.

Our hope is that the half-dozen key outcomes noted have convinced you of the importance of the research—ours and that of many others—to not-for-profits in our sectors. We believe that partnerships with the private sector are a reality of the future and a necessity in certain cases given our current climate and the forecasted reality of North American society in the coming decades. The book has shared *The Partnership Protocol*, a clear, industry-built process to help not-for-profits engage responsibly in partnerships with the private sector. The book shares the input of experts from related domains, illustrative case studies, and important literature. We are confident in its detail and encourage you to use it to make your partnerships long lasting, beneficial to all partners, and responsible to the society in which we all live.

GLOSSARY

activation—Investment by the parties above and beyond the rights fees to promote the association, reach target markets, and increase the image transfer process (strategies that the sponsor or sponsee funds in addition to what was outlined in the contract and then implements to increase the effectiveness of the sponsorship).

benefactor—The target population, groups, or individuals who benefit from the partnership's objectives.

capacity imbalance—The relative strengths and weaknesses in relation to the capacity of each partner. Note that the capacity of each partner does not have to be equal because each partner can bring resources or skills that the other partner lacks.

cause marketing—The integration of a cause or charitable initiative into the marketing plan or program of an organization. Cause marketing is common today in event marketing in which any event from a 5K run to a professional sport club activity has a charity and an accompanying fund-raising effort associated with it. The organization then includes the cause in its marketing activities around the event to improve its brand image and attract interest.

champion—A person to lead communications to stakeholders and showcase the partnered project.

change order—A clear process to approve changes to a partnership.

clawback—A requirement to pay some or all of the received benefits if performance objectives are not achieved; penalties can diminish with time until the expiration of a lease, according to the negotiated contract.

collaborative partnerships—The collaboration of efforts and input, usually in the form of a longer-term commitment, from both the public and private sphere, resulting in the cocreation of mutually beneficial outcomes.

communication strategy—A plan to build and share information both internally (to partners) and externally (to broader society).

consumer perceptions—The perceptions of consumers or audiences about a particular brand, service, or partnership.

corporate social responsibility—Often dubbed CSR, it refers to a private-sector organization (corporation) that invests resources, effort, and time into improving its local city, province or state, country, and planet in an effort to give back.

credibility—Public confidence or belief in the goals and objectives of the partnership.

culturally appropriate—Designing programs and campaigns with an aware-ness of their appeal to diverse cultural groups (e.g., taking into account language, religion, and traditional values).

employee volunteering—Volunteering by employees of a certain organization for a particular cause, usually related to the organization's brand or mission.

exclusivity—The right given to a sponsor to be the only sponsor of a given event in their business category (e.g., automobile, airline). Also called category exclusivity to emphasize the ownership of a specific category.

feedback loop—Information flow from partnership to target and target back to partners to help monitor and assess strengths and weaknesses, expecta-tions, and barriers to generate the most favorable outcomes.

funding partner—Partners who are established for their ability to provide financial support.

gatekeeper—A person or group who holds access to the desired target group.

image transfer—A key element in understanding how sponsorship works, image transfer is considered in the sponsor–sponsee association, whereby the transfer of some image from one party to another occurs in the minds of the target audience. Image transfer is often the objective of a sponsor or private-sector partner when seeking a partnership with a not-for-profit organization.

image values—The way that an organization perceives itself and would like others (consumers) to perceive their goods or services. Can also be used to represent the current reality of how consumers view a certain organization.

implementing partner—A partner who is established or sought for their ability to provide support in achieving and maintaining the partnership's goals and objectives.

inactivity crisis—An important social challenge in the United States, Canada, and other developed countries of the world, the inactivity crisis refers to the declining rates of fitness, sport participation, and physical activity partici-pation in males and females of all ages, leading to, some argue, mounting incidence of chronic disease and increasing health care costs.

legacy—The enduring benefits that will remain for both partners after the partnership ends. In major partnerships, such as those for an Olympic Games, legacy takes on increased importance.

megaevent—A large-scale national or international sporting event that typi-cally involves multiple partnerships and financial and community support from the local region associated with it. Examples include the Super Bowl, Olympic Games, Grey Cup, and Masters.

micro-philanthropy—A small-scale funding agreement or donation.

nonfinancial support—Nonmonetary resources that support a partnership, often called value-in-kind (VIK) or contra. They can be products or services. Examples include volunteers, food, beverages, equipment, media time, and word-of-mouth effort.

outcome indicators—The specified indicators of a partnership's success, fail-ures, and conclusion. These are typically agreed upon jointly by the partners.

The Partnership Protocol—Developed by a steering committee of academic, government, business, and not-for-profit experts, this document provides guidance to build, manage, and evaluate sport participation, public health, and physical activity partnerships.

partnership—Denotes a relationship between organizations or stakeholders. Partnerships can be in multiple forms between two or more businesses, charities, sport organizations, community groups, local government offices, and other forms of organizations.

performance monitoring—Daily, weekly, monthly, or quarterly monitoring of the performance of the partnership in achieving its goals and objectives.

philanthropic linkage—Donations of money, time, or goods from a private enterprise to a public (usually charitable) organization or event.

power balance—Mutual understanding of the hierarchy of power, benefits, and risks between partners.

private partner—A for-profit, generally corporate organization who operates independently of government and whose goals are based on providing return to shareholders, typically by revenue generation or brand enhancement. Private partner organizations include business retailers, manufacturers, service providers, professional sport teams, and media.

public partner—A not-for-profit or charity organization (e.g., KidsHealth, United States Triathlon Association, Hockey Canada), a multisport organization (e.g., United States Olympic Committee, Commonwealth Games Canada, World Anti-Doping Agency), a health organization involved in physical activity (e.g., World Health Organization), or a government department (e.g., Health Canada, Sport Canada) that funds sport participation, public health, or physical activity organizations.

public–private partnership—Also known as a PPP, a strategic initiative between a public (not-for-profit) organization and a private (for-profit) organization. In some cases PPPs involve more than two partners and can involve many.

responsiveness—A planned approach to consider necessary changes in a partnership in response to monitoring and evaluation of its performance.

role model—A person, worth imitating, who leads by example and influences another's development through his or her ability to be a powerful teacher of knowledge, skills, and values.

shared risk—Risks assumed by both the public and private partner in establishing and maintaining the partnership.

social compatibility—The level of congruency between the partners' organizational values and cultures.

social media—The use of Internet technology for social exchanges of news and information (e.g., blogs, Twitter).

spillover benefits—Benefits that are beyond the original scope of the partnership, including increases in tourism, job creation, and regional economic development.

sport—Forms of play and recreation; organized, casual, or competitive sport; and indigenous sports or games.

stakeholders—Individuals, groups, and affiliated entities that influence, use, or promote the partnership's goals, purpose, and objectives. The "big three" stakeholder groups in partnerships include government, public organizations, and nongovernmental organizations.

storytelling—Publically sharing information about the partnership (or other activity) to all stakeholders before, during, and after the partnership. Note that storytelling can be internal (to employees and stakeholders) and external (to customers and the public).

third party—An organization external to the two partnering organizations that provides support or resources to help the partnership be realized (e.g., agency, event management firm, industry association, advocate).

tools of inactivity—Consumer goods that increase the practice of sedentary leisure activities (e.g., televisions, video games, personal computing, and portable electronic devices).

transparency—Open and easily accessible disclosure of purpose, objectives, influences, partners, and sources and uses of funds.

trust dynamics—The level of confidence and mutual trust between partners.

REFERENCES

Active Healthy Kids Canada. 2009. *Report card on physical activity for children and youth.* Retrieved from www.activehealthykids.ca.

Altheide, D.L. 1987. Ethnographic content analysis. *Qualitative Sociology* 10:65–77.

Andersen, L.B., P. Schnchr, M. Schroll, et al. 2000. All-cause mortality associated with physical activity during leisure time, work, sports and cycling to work. *Archives of Internal Medicine* 160:1621–1628.

Andranovich, G., M.J. Burbank, and C.H. Heying. 2001. Olympic cities: Lessons learned from mega-event politics. *Journal of Urban Affairs* 23 (2): 113.

Armstrong, J. Scott. 2010. *Persuasive advertising.* London: Palgrave Macmillan.

Ayer, S. 2010. *Insights for strategic corporate fundraising: Further findings from the Canada Survey of Business Contributions to Community.* Toronto: Imagine Canada.

Ayer, S. 2011. Interview by author, Sudbury, ON, May 31.

Ayer, S. 2011. *Corporate giving in Canada: The latest data, trends, and implications.* Conference presentation at the Imagine Canada Business Community Partnership Forum.

Ayer, S., M. Hall, and L. Vodarek. 2009. *Perspectives on fundraising: What charities report to the Canada Revenue Agency.* Toronto: Imagine Canada.

Babiak, K. 2007. Determinants of interorganizational relationships: The case of a Canadian nonprofit sport organization. *Journal of Sport Management* 21:338–376.

Babiak, K., and L. Thibault. 2009. Challenges in multiple cross-sector partnerships. *Nonprofit and Voluntary Sector Quarterly* 38: 117–143.

Barr, D.A. 2007. A research protocol to evaluate the effectiveness of public–private partnerships as a means to improve health and welfare systems worldwide. *American Journal of Public Health* 97 (1): 19–25.

Beaulac, J., Olavarria, M., and Kristjansson, E. 2010. A Community-Based Hip-Hop Dance Program for Youth in a Disadvantaged Community in Ottawa: Implementation Findings, *Health Promotion Practice,* 11(3), 61-69.

Bekkers, R., and P. Wiepking. 2010. A literature review of empirical studies of philanthropy: Eight mechanisms that drive charitable giving. *Nonprofit & Voluntary Sector Quarterly.* 40(5): 924-973.

Berger, I., O'Reilly, N., Parent, M., Seguin, B., and Hernandez, T. 2008. Determinants of Sport Participation Among Canadian Adolescents, *Sport Management Review,* 11(3), 277-307.

Bingham, T., and M. Conner. 2010. *The new social learning: A guide to transforming organizations through social media.* San Francisco: Berrett-Koehler.

Bloom, M., Grant, M., & Watt, D. 2005. *Strengthening Canada: The socio-economic benefits of sport participation in Canada.* Ottawa, Canada: The Conference Board of Canada,.

Boone, T. 2004. Is sports nutrition for sale? *Professionalization of Exercise Physiology* 7 (7). Retrieved from http://faculty.css.edu/tboone2/asep/ Is SportsNutritionForSale.html.

Boston College Center for Corporate Citizenship. 2011. *Cause related marketing.* Retrieved from www.bcccc.net/index.cfm?fuseaction=page.viewPage&pageID=2102&nodeID=1.

Bryant, C., J. Lindenberger, C. Brown, E. Kent, J.M. Schreiber, M. Bustillo, and M.W. Canright. 2001. A social marketing approach to increasing enrollment in a public health program: A case study of the Texas WIC program. *Human organization* 60 (3): 234-246.

Bryson, J.M., B.C. Crosby, M.M. Stone, & J.C. Mortenson. 2008. *Collaboration in fighting traffic congestion: A study of Minnesota's urban partnership agreement.* Hubert H. Humphrey Institute of Public Affairs, University of Minnesota.

Bryson, J.M., B.C. Crosby, and M.M. Stone. 2006. The design and implementation of cross- sector collaborations: Propositions from the literature. *Public Administration Review* 66:44–55.

Buunk, A.P., J.M. Peiro, and C. Griffioen. 2007. A positive role model may stimulate career-oriented behavior. *Journal of Applied Social Psychology* 37:1489–1500.

Buse, K., and A. Waxman 2001. Public–private health partnerships: A strategy for WHO. *Bulletin of the World Health Organization* 79 (8).

Butterworth, T. 2011. ABC News attacks scientist who exposed bias in obesity research. *Forbes.* Retrieved from www.forbes.com/sites/trevorbutterworth/2011/06/22/abc-news-attacks-scientist-who-exposed-bias-in-obesity-research/.

Canadian Sponsorship Landscape Study (CSLS). 2011. *5th annual.* Retrieved from www. sponsorshiplandscape.ca.

Carroll, A. 1999. Corporate social responsibility: Evolution of a definitional construct. *Business and Society* 28 (3): 268–295.

Charities Directorate. 2010. *Strategic directions exercise.* Ottawa, ON: Charities Directorate.

Cheadle, A., R. Egger, J.P. LoGerfo, J. Walwick, and S. Schwartz. 2010. A community-organizing approach to promoting physical activity in older adults: The Southeast senior physical activity network. *Health Promotion Practice* 11: 197–204.

CMHL. 2009. *Canadian Multicultural Hockey League: Latest news.* Retrieved from www.cmhl.ca/newsdesk/index.php.

Coady, M. 2007. *Giving in numbers 2007 edition.* New York: Committee Encouraging Corporate Philanthropy.

Coady, M. 2009. *Giving in numbers 2009 edition.* New York: Committee Encouraging Corporate Philanthropy.

Colley, R.C., D. Garriguet, I. Janssen, C.L. Craig, J. Clarke, and M.S. Tremblay. 2011. Physical activity levels of Canadian adults: Results from the 2007–2009 Canadian Health Measures Survey. *Health Reports* 22 (1): 7–24.

Committee Encouraging Corporate Philanthropy (CECP). 2009. *Business's social contract. Capturing the corporate philanthropy opportunity.* Retrieved from www.corporatephilanthropy.org/pdfs/research_reports/SocialContract.pdf.

Commonwealth Games Canada. 2009. *Application tool for partnership filter.* Retrieved from www. sportanddev.org/toolkit/?uNewsID=116.

Cornwell, T.B., S.W. Pruitt, and J.M. Clark. 2005. The relationship between major-league sports' official sponsorship announcements and the stock prices of sponsoring firms. *Journal of the Academy of Marketing Science* 33 (4): 401–412.

Cote, L. & Leclere, H. 2000. How clinical teachers perceive the doctor-patient relationship and themselves as role models, Academic Medicine, 75, pp. 1117-1124.

Cousens, L., M. Barnes, J. Stevens, C. Mallen, and C. Bradish. 2006. Who's your partner? Who's your ally? Exploring the characteristics of public, private, and voluntary recreation linkages. *Journal of Park & Recreation Administration* 24 (1): 32–55.

Crabbe, T. 2000. A sporting chance? Using sport to tackle drug use and crime. *Drugs: Education, Prevention and Policy* 7:381–391.

Craig, C.L., C. Tudor-Locke, and A. Bauman. 2007. Twelve-month effects of Canada on the Move: A population-wide campaign to promote pedometer use and walking. *Health Education Research* 22 (3): 406–413.

Crompton, J. 2004. Conceptualization and alternate operationalizations of the measurement of sponsorship effectiveness in sport. *Leisure Studies,* 23(3), 267-281.

Cruess, S.R., R.L. Cruess, and Y. Steinert. 2008. Role modelling—making the most of a powerful teaching strategy. *British Medical Journal* 336 (7646): 718–721.

Dart, R., and B. Zimmerman. 2000. After government cuts: Insights from two Ontario "enterprising nonprofits." In K. Banting (ed.), *The nonprofit sector in Canada: Roles and relationships* (pp. 107–148). Kingston, ON: School of Policy Studies, Queen's University.

Dharod, J.M., R. Drewette-Card, and D. Crawford. 2011. Development of the Oxford Hills Healthy Moms Project using a social marketing process: A community-based physical activity and nutrition intervention for low-socioeconomic-status mothers in a rural area in Maine. *Health Promotion Practice* 12:312–321.

Dixon, J., C. Sindall, and C. Banwell. 2004. Exploring the intersectoral partnerships guiding Australia's dietary advice. *Health Promotion International* 19(1). Oxford University Press.

Drumwright, M.E. 1996. Company advertising with a social dimension: The role of non-economic criteria. *Journal of Marketing* 60 (4): 71–87.

Easwaramoorthy, M., C. Barr, G. Gumulka, and L. Hartford,. 2006. *Business support for charities and nonprofits*. Toronto: Imagine Canada.

Fahy, J., F. Farrelly, and P. Quester. 2004. Competitive advantage through sponsorship. *European Journal of Marketing* 38 (8): 1013–1030.

Farag, J., and L. Brittain. 2009. Sports in the public–private arena: City of Toronto. *Government Finance Review* 25 (3): 73–76.

Ferk, B., and P. Ferk. 2008. Public–private partnership in Slovenia: An analysis of one of the first successful projects of public–private partnership in Slovenia—the Stožice Stadium. *European Public Private Partnership Law Review* 3 (4): 175–184.

Forzani Group. 2009. *Our partnerships: Hockey Canada*. Retrieved from www.forzanigroup.com/ourPartnerships.aspx?selected=hockeycanada.

Foster, M.K., A.G. Meinhard, I.E. Berger, and P. Krpan. 2009. Corporate philanthropy in the Canadian context: From damage control to improving society. *Nonprofit and Voluntary Sector Quarterly* 38: 441-466.

Foundation Center. 2011. *Distribution of grants by field-specific recipient type and foundation type, circa 2009*. New York: Foundation Center.

Freedhoff, Y., and P. Hébert. 2011. Partnerships between health organizations and the food industry risk derailing public health nutrition. *Canadian Medical Association Journal*, DOI:10.1503/cmaj.110085.

Frisby, W., L. Thibault, and L. Kikulis. 2004. The organizational dynamics of under-managed partnerships in leisure service departments. *Leisure Studies* 23 (2): 109–112.

Gierl, H., and A. Kirchner. 1999. Emotionale bindung und imagetransfer durch sportsponsoring. *Werbeforschung & Praxis* 44 (3): 32–35.

Gifts in Kind International. 2008. *Gifts in Kind International annual report*. Retrieved from http://about.good360.org/images/pdfs/2007_gik_annual_report.pdf.

Gilmore, A. 2004. Local cultural strategies: A strategic review. *Cultural Trends* 13 (51): 3–32.

Giving USA Foundation. 2011. *Giving USA 2011: The annual report on philanthropy for the year 2010*. Retrieved from www.givingusareports.org.

Good360. 2011. *Quick facts about us*. Retrieved from http://about.good360.org/contents/49.

Googins, B., V. Veleva, C. Pinney, P. Mirvis, R. Carapinha, and R. Raffaelli. 2009. *State of corporate citizenship 2009: Weathering the storm*. Chestnut Hill, MA: Boston College Center for Corporate Citizenship.

Grier, S., and C.A. Bryant. 2005. Social marketing in public health *Annual Review of Public Health* 26:319–339.

Gwinner, K.P., and J. Eaton. 1999. Building brand image through event sponsorship: The role of image transfer. *Journal of Advertising* 28 (4): 47–57.

Hall, H. 2009. Corporate and individual giving: What to expect in coming months. *Chronicle of philanthropy*. Retrieved from http://philanthropy.com/premium/articles/v21/i09/09001001.htm.

Hall, M., A. Andrukow, C. Barr, K. Brock, M. De Wit, D. Embuldeniya, et al. 2003. *The capacity to serve: A qualitative study of the challenges facing Canada's nonprofit and voluntary organizations*. Toronto: Canadian Centre for Philanthropy.

Hall, M.H., M. de Wit, D. Lasby, D. McIver, T. Evers, C. Johnston, et al. 2005. *Cornerstones of community: Highlights of the National Survey of Nonprofit and Voluntary Organizations*. Ottawa, ON: Statistics Canada.

Hall, M., D. Lasby, S. Ayer, and W.D. Gibbons. 2009. *Caring Canadians, involved Canadians. Highlights from the 2007 Canada Survey of Giving, Volunteering, and Participating*. Ottawa, ON: Statistics Canada.

Healthy Kids, Healthy Schools. 2009. *Healthy Kids, Healthy Schools Organization*. Retrieved from www.healthykidshealthyschools.org/projects/.

Hersey, J., B. Kelly, A. Roussel, L. Curtis, J. Horne, P. Williams-Piehota, S. Kuester, and R. Farris. 2012. The value of partnerships in state obesity prevention and control programs, *Health Promot Pract* 13(2): 222-229.

Hockey Canada. 2009. *Hockey Canada corporate partnerships*. Retrieved from www.hockeycanada.ca/index.php/ci_id/ 6839/la_id/1.htm.

Hodge, G., and C. Greve. 2007. Public–private partnerships: An international performance review. *Public Administration Review* 67 (3): 545–558.

Hoek, J., and P. Gendall, P. 2002. When do ex-sponsors become ambush marketers? *International Journal of Sports Marketing & Sponsorship* 3 (4): 383–402.

Holland, L. 2003. Can the principle of the ecological footprint be applied to measure the environmental sustainability of business? *Corporate Social Responsibility and Environmental Management* 10 (4): 224–233.

Homeless World Cup. 2009. *The Homeless World Cup Organisation*. Retrieved from www.homelessworldcup.org/.

Houpt, S. 2011. In sunny Riviera, storm clouds gather. *Globe and Mail*, June 24.

Hurvid, D., Ayer, S., Ellison, D. 2011. *Foundation insights*. Conference presentation at Imagine Canada's Business Community Partnership Forum.

IEG. 2011. Sponsorship spending: 2010 proves better than expected; bigger gains set for 2011. Retrieved from http://sponsorship.com

Innes, J.E., and D.E. Booher. 1999. Consensus building and complex adaptive systems: A framework for evaluating collaborative planning. *Journal of the American Planning Association* 65 (4): 412–423.

Internet World Stats. 2012. *Internet world stats: Usage and population statistics*. Retrieved from www.internetworldstats.com.

Irwin, R.L., T. Lachowetz, T.B. Cornwell, and J.S. Clark. 2003. Cause-related sport sponsorship: An assessment of spectator beliefs, attitudes and behavioural intentions. *Sport Marketing Quarterly* 12 (3): 131–139.

Jacobson, C., and S. Ok Choi. 2008. Success factors: Public works and public–private partnerships. *International Journal of Public Sector Management* 21 (6): 637–657.

Joyner, K. 2007. Dynamic evolution in public–private partnerships: The role of key actors in managing multiple stakeholders. *Managerial Law* 49 (5/6): 206–217.

Kao, A. 2008. *The 2007 contributions report*. The Conference Board. Retrieved from www.conferenceboard.ca/documents.aspx?did=2427.

Katzmarzyk, P.T., and I. Janssen. 2004. The economic costs associated with physical inactivity and obesity in Canada: An update. *Canadian Journal of Applied Physiology* 29 (1): 90–115.

Kennedy, S., and M.S. Rosentraub. 2000. Public–private partnerships, professional sports teams, and the protection of the public's interests. *American Review of Public Administration* 30 (4): 436–459.

Kicking AIDS Out. 2008. *The network: Overview*. Retrieved from www.kickingaidsout.net/WhatISKickingAIDSOut/ Sider/TheNetwork.aspx.

Kids in Action. 2003. *Fitness for Children: Birth to Age 5*. http://www.aahperd.org/naspe/publications/teachingTools/upload/brochure.pdf

Kozinets, R.V. 2002. The field behind the screen: Using netnography for marketing research in online communities. *Journal of Marketing Research* 39:61-72.

Kraak, V.I., S.K. Kumanyika, and M. Story. 2009. The commercial marketing of healthy lifestyles to address the global child and adolescent obesity pandemic: Prospects, pitfalls and priorities. *Public Health Nutrition* 12:2027–2036.

Kruger, J., K. Nelson, P. Klein, L.E. McCurdy, P. Pride, and J.C. Andy. 2011. Building on partnerships: Reconnecting kids with nature for health benefits. *Health Promotion Practice* 11: 340-346.

Lawrence, S., and R. Mukai. 2011. *Foundation growth and giving estimates: Current outlook* (2011 ed.). New York: Foundation Center.

Lindsey, I., and D. Banda. 2011. Sport and the fight against HIV/AIDS in Zambia: A "partnership approach." *International Review for the Sociology of Sport* 46:90–107.

Lornic, J. 2010. Small donations big deal for local sports. *Globe and Mail*. August 12.

Love, T. 2006. Corporate philanthropy: Getting it right; corporate philanthropists engage both their head and their heart. *New Zealand Management* 53(9).

Maher, A., N. Wilson, L. Signal, and G. Thomson. 2006. Patterns of sport sponsorship by gambling, alcohol and food companies: An Internet survey. *BMC Public Health* 6:95–99.

Mainwaring, S. 2011. *How non-profits and brands partner for social capital*. Retrieved from We First Blog, June 14.

Margolis, J.D., Anger Elfenbein, H., and Walsh, J.P. 2007. *Does It Pay To Be Good? A Meta-Analysis and Redirection of Research on the Relationship Between Corporate Social and Financial Performance, working paper*, July 26: http://stakeholder.bu.edu/Docs/Walsh,%20Jim%20Does%20It%20Pay%20to%20Be%20Good.pdf

Marks, J.H. and Thompson, D.B. 2011. Shifting the Focus: Conflict of Interest and the Food Industry, *The American Journal of Bioethics*, 11(1), 44-46.

Marx, D. M., Ko, S. J., & Friedman, R. A. 2009. The "Obama effect": How a salient role model reduces race-based performance differences. *Journal of Experimental Social Psychology*, 45, 953-956.

Marx, D.M., and J.S. Roman. 2002. Female role models: Protecting women's math test performance. *Personality and Social Psychology Bulletin* 28:1183–1193.

Matsudo, S.M., and V.R. Matsudo. 2006. Coalitions and networks: Facilitating global physical activity promotion. *International Journal of Health Promotion & Education*: 133–138.

Meier, M., and M. Saavedra. 2009. Esther Phiri and the Moutawakel effect in Zambia: An analysis of the use of female role models in sport-for-development. *Sport in Society: Cultures, Commerce, Media, Politics* 12 (9): 1158–1176.

Melanson, A. 2011. *The ABCs of RBC's philanthropic focus*. Bloom for Nonprofits. Retrieved from http://bloomfornonprofits.com/2011/02/the-abcs-of-rbc%E2%80%99s-philanthropic-focus/.

Misener, K., and A. Doherty. 2009. A case study of organizational capacity in nonprofit community sport. *Journal of Sport Management* 23 (4): 457–482.

Mohr, L.A., and D.J. Webb. 2005. The effects of corporate social responsibility on price and consumer responses. *Journal of Consumer Affairs* 39 (1): 121–147.

Muirhead, S.A. 2006. *Philanthropy and business the changing agenda*. New York: The Conference Board.

Murumets, K., N. O'Reilly, M.S. Tremblay, and P.T. Katzmarzyk. 2010. Public private partnerships in physical activity and sport: Principles for successful, responsible, partnerships. Symposium.

National Center for Charitable Statistics. 2011. *Registered nonprofit organizations by major purpose or activity (NTEE code = sports and recreation)*. The Urban Institute, National Center for Charitable Statistics. Retrieved from http://nccsdataweb.urban.org/.

Nicholls, J.A.F., S. Roslow, and S. Dublish. 1999. Brand recall and brand preference at sponsored golf and tennis tournaments. *European Journal of Marketing* 33 (3/4): 365–386.

Nike. 2004, October 20. *Nike names new VP of corporate responsibility, Maria Eitel becomes president of the Nike Foundation*. Retrieved from www.csrwire.com/press/press_release/ 24945-Nike-Names-New-VP-of-Corporate-Responsibility-Maria-Eitel-Becomes-President-of-the-Nike-Foundation.

Nike. 2007, December 11. *Nike and Ashoka's Changemakers launched "Sport for a Better World Competition" at Next Step 2007*. Retrieved from www.prlog.org/10041524-nike-and-ashoka-changemakers-launched-sport-for-better-world-competition-at-next-step-2007.html.

Nike. 2008a. *Nike Foundation*. Retrieved from www.nikefoundation.org/.

Nike. 2008b, October 17. *Nike Gamechangers: The lowdown*. Retrieved from http://inside.nike.com/ blogs/gamechangers-en_US/2008/10/25/gamechangers-converge-on-s-o-paulo-to-change-the-world.

Nike. 2009. *Nike & CARE support Kenyan youth soccer*. Retrieved from www.nikebiz.com/responsibility/ community_programs /features/KASE_soccer.html.

Njaul, R.J.A., F.W. Mosha, and D. De Savigny. 2009. Case studies in public-private-partnership in health with the focus of enhancing the accessibility of health interventions. *Tanzania Journal of Health Research* 11 (4): 235–249.

Olshansky, S.J., D.J. Passaro, R.C. Hershow, J. Layden, B.A. Carnes, J. Brody, L. Hayflick, R.N. Butler, D.B. Allison, and D.S. Ludwig. 2005. A potential decline in life expectancy in the United States in the 21st century. *New England Journal of Medicine* 352:1138–1145.

Ontario Parks. 2011. Learn to Camp at Ontario Parks. Retrieved from www.ontarioparks.com/ learntocamp/online_resources.html.

O'Reilly, N., M. Lyberger, L. McCarthy, B. Seguin, and J. Nadeau. 2008. Mega-special-event promotions and intent-to-purchase: A longitudinal analysis of the Super Bowl. *Journal of Sport Management* 22 (4): 392–409.

O'Reilly, N. 2010. *Public–private partnerships in the sport and physical activity contexts*. A literature review completed as a precursor to this project. Available from ParticipACTION.

O'Reilly, N., and G. Foster. 2010. *Not for profit / private sector partnerships in sport and physical activity: ParticipACTION as champion*. Stanford Graduate School of Business, Case SPM 43.

O'Reilly, N., and J. Madill. 2009. Methods and metrics in sponsorship evaluation. *Journal of Sponsorship* 2 (3): 215–230.

Pagdadis, S.A., Sorett, S.M., Rapaport, F.M., Edmonds, C.J., Rafshoon, G.S., & Hale, M.L. 2008. A road map to success for public–private partnerships of public infrastructure initiatives. *Journal of Public Equity* 8–18.

Parent, M.M., and J. Harvey. 2009. Towards a management model for sport and physical activity community-based partnerships. *European Sport Management Quarterly* 9 (1): 23–45.

ParticipACTION. 2009. *Annual report 2009*. Retrieved from www.ParticipACTION.com/ AnnualReport/index.html.

ParticipACTION. 2010. *The Partnership Protocol*. Retrieved from www.participaction.com/ wp-content/uploads/2012/10/partnershipprotocol_english_final.pdf.

Pegoraro, A.L., S.M. Ayer, and N.J. O'Reilly. 2010. Consumer consumption and advertising through sport. *American Behavioral Scientist* 53:1454–1475.

Pham, M.T., and G.V. Johar. 2001. Market prominence biases in sponsor identification: Processes and consequentiality. *Psychology and Marketing* 18 (2): 123–143.

Pitter, R. 2009. Finding the Kieran way: Recreational sport, health, and environmental policy in Nova Scotia. *Journal of Sport & Social Issues* 33 (3): 331–351.

Pound, R.W. 1996. The importance of commercialism for the Olympic Movement. *International Olympic Committee: Olympic Message* 3:10–13.

RBC. 2011. *Donations*. Retrieved from www.rbc.com/donations/.

Rifon, N.J., S.M. Choi, C.S. Trimble, and H. Li. 2004. Congruence effects in sponsorship. *Journal of Advertising* 33 (1): 29–42.

Right To Play. 2009. *When children play, the world wins*. Retrieved from www.righttoplay.com.

Right To Play. 2008a. Sport and health: Preventing disease and promoting health (chapter 1). In *Harnessing the power of sport for development and peace: Recommendations to governments*. Toronto: Sport for Development and Peace International Working Group.

Right To Play. 2008b. Developing effective policies and programs (chapter 7). In *Harnessing the power of sport for development and peace: Recommendations to governments*. Toronto: Sport for Development and Peace International Working Group.

Robins, F. 2005. The future of corporate social responsibility. *Asian Business & Management* 4 (2): 95–115.

Rosentraub, M., and D. Swindell. 2009. Of devils and details: Bargaining for successful public/ private partnerships between cities and sports teams. *Public Administration Quarterly* 33 (1): 118–148.

Rowe et al. 2009. Funding food science and nutrition research: Financial conflicts and scientific integrity. *American Journal of Clinical Nutrition* 89:1–7.

Roy, D.P. 2008. Impact of new minor league baseball stadiums on game attendance. *Sport Marketing Quarterly* 17 (3): 146–153.

Sagalyn, L.B. 2007. Private/public development: Lessons from history, research, and practice. *Journal of the American Planning Association* 73 (1): 7–22.

Saikaly, E. 2009. Personal correspondence with author. January 15, 2009.

Salamon, L.M. 1995. *Partners in public service: Government–nonprofit relations in the modern welfare state.* Baltimore: John Hopkins University Press.

Scherer, J., and M. Sam. 2008. Public consultation and stadium developments: Coercion and the polarization of debate. *Sociology of Sport Journal* 25 (4): 443–461.

Scott, K. 2003. *Funding matters: The impact of Canada's new funding regime on nonprofit and voluntary organizations.* Ottawa, ON: Canadian Council on Social Development.

Seguin, B., M. Lyberger, N. O'Reilly, and L. McCarthy. 2005. Internationalizing ambush marketing: The Olympic brand and country of origin. *International Journal of Sport Sponsorship and Marketing* 6 (4): 216–230.

Seguin, B., and N. O'Reilly. 2007. Sponsorship in the trenches: Case study evidence of its legitimate place in the promotional mix. *Sport Journal* 10 (1).

Seguin, B., M. Parent, and N. O'Reilly. 2010. Corporate support: A corporate social responsibility alternative to traditional event sponsorship. *International Journal of Sport Management and Marketing* 7 (3/4): 202–222.

Shields, M., M.D. Carroll, and C.L. Ogden. 2011. Adult obesity prevalence in Canada and the United States. *NCHS Data Brief,* no. 56. Hyattsville, MD: National Center for Health Statistics.

Shields, M., M.S. Tremblay, M. Laviolette, C.L. Craig, I. Janssen, and S. Connor Gorber. 2010. Fitness of Canadian adults: Results from the 2007–2009 Canadian Health Measures Survey. *Health Reports* 21 (1): 21–36.

Shirky, C. 2010. *Cognitive surplus: Creativity and generosity in a connected age.* New York: Penguin Group.

Siegfried, J., and A. Zimbalist. 2000. The economics of sports facilities and their communities. *Journal of Economic Perspectives* 14 (3): 95–114.

Simon, M. 2011. 2011, July 27. *Obesity panacea blog.* Retrieved from http://blogs.plos.org/ obesitypanacea/2011/07/19/we-need-to-stop-arranging-society-around-ridiculous-choices.

Sport and Development. 2009a. *About this platform.* Retrieved from www.sportanddev.org/ about_this_platform/.

Sport and Development. 2009b. *Partnerships.* Retrieved from www.sportanddev.org/ toolkit/ partnerships/.

Starkman, R. 2009. *Canadian Olympians stand by charity.* Retrieved from www.thestar.com/Sports/ article/587624. February 14.

Statistics Canada. 2010. Sport participation in Canada, 2005. *Culture, Tourism and the Centre for Education Statistics.* Vol. Catalogue no. 81-595-MIE—No. 060: Statistics Canada XPE, Health Reports, Vol. 21, no. 1, March.

Steger, and Parsons. 2006. *Exploring corporate philanthropy.* Committee to Encourage Corporate Philanthropy (CECP). New York. Retrieved from www.corporatephilanthropy.org/pdfs/ research_reports/ExploringCorpPhil.pdf.

ThinkFirst. 2009. *Programs.* Retrieved from www.thinkfirst.ca/programs/index.aspx.

Today's Parent. 2009. Healthy Kids 2009. Retrieved from www.todaysparent.com/healthykids/article. jsp?content =20081205_164559_9768&page=1.

Trafford, S., and T. Proctor. 2006. Successful joint venture partnerships: Public–private partnerships. *International Journal of Public Sector Management* 19 (2): 117–129.

Tremblay, M. 2011. Public-private sector partnerships in physical activity and sport: Principles for successful, resposible partnerships: *The Partnership Protocol.* 2011 Canadian Obesity Summit, Montreal, Canada.

Tremblay, M.S., J.D. Barnes, J.L. Copeland, and D.W. Esliger. 2005. Conquering childhood inactivity: Is the answer in the past? *Medicine and Science in Sports and Exercise* 37:1187–1194.

Tremblay, M.S., M. Shields, M. Laviolette, C.L. Craig, I. Janssen, and S. Connor Gorber. 2010. Fitness of Canadian children and youth: Results from the 2007–2009 Canadian Health Measures Survey. *Health Reports* 21 (1): 7–20.

Tremblay, M.S., and C.L. Craig. 2009. ParticipACTION: Overview and introduction of baseline research on the "new" ParticipACTION. *International Journal of Behavioral Nutrition and Physical Activity* 6:84.

Tremblay, M.S., R. Colley, T.J. Saunders, G.N. Healy, and N. Owen. 2010. Physiological and health implications of a sedentary lifestyle. *Applied Physiology, Nutrition and Metabolism* 35:725–740.

Tremblay, M.S., D.W. Esliger, J.L. Copeland, J.D. Barnes, and D.R. Bassett. 2008. Moving forward by looking back: Lessons learned from lost lifestyles. *Applied Physiology, Nutrition and Metabolism* 33:836–842.

Tremblay, M.S., P.T. Katzmarzyk, and J.D. Willms. 2002. Temporal trends in overweight and obesity in Canada, 1981–1996. *International Journal of Obesity and Related Metabolic Disorders* 26 (4): 538–543.

Tremblay, M.S., M. Shields, M. Laviolette, C.L. Craig, I. Janssen, and S. Connor Gorber. 2010. Fitness of Canadian children and youth: Results from the 2007–2009 Canadian Health Measures Survey. *Health Reports* 21 (1): 7–20.

United Nations. 2007. *Guiding principles for public–private collaboration for humanitarian action.* Retrieved from www.undg.org/docs/10472/guiding-principles-for-public-private-partnerships.pdf.

Vail, S. 2007. Community development and sport participation. *Journal of Sport Management* 21 (4): 571-596.

van Kempen, P.P. 2008. *Wake up! Unleash the potential of partnerships between companies and NGOs.* Retrieved from www.sportanddev.org/toolkit/partnerships /two_step_by_step_guides_ for_ngos/.

Varadarajan, P.R., and Menon, A. 1988. Cause-related marketing: A coalignment of marketing strategy and corporate philanthropy. *Journal of Marketing* 52:58–74.

Vining, A.R., and A.E. Boardman. 2008. Public–private partnerships in Canada: Theory and evidence. *Canadian Public Administration* 51 (1): 9–44.

Waldie, P. 2011 (March 25). Tax-rule changes take charities by surprise. *Globe and Mail.*

Waters, R. D., Burke, K. A., Jackson, Z. H., and Buning, J. D. 2011. Using stewardship to cultivate fandom online: comparing how National Football League teams use their web sites and Facebook to engage their fans. *International Journal of Sport Communication,* 4(2), 163-177.Website Optimization. com. n.d. *World wide Internet report.* www.websiteoptimization.com/bw/1103/.

Webster's Online Dictionary. 2012. Retrieved from www.webster-dictionary.org/.

Weiermair, K., M. Peters, and J. Frehse. 2008. Success factors for public private partnership: Cases in alpine tourism development. *Journal of Services Research* 8:7–21.

Weir, M. 2009. *The Mike Weir Foundation: About us.* Retrieved from www.themikeweirfoundation. com/about-us.

Wettenhall, R. 2003. The rhetoric and reality of public–private partnerships. *Public Organization Review: A Global Journal* 3:77-107.

Widdus, R. 2001. Public–private partnerships for health: Their main targets, their diversity, and their future directions. *Bulletin of the World Health Organization* 79:713–720.

Wing, K.T., K.L. Roeger, and T.H. Pollak. 2011. *The nonprofit sector in brief. Public charities, giving, and volunteering, 2010.* Washington, DC: The Urban Institute.

Wood, L., R. Snelgrove, and K. Danylchuk. 2010. Segmenting volunteer charity fundraisers using identity theory. *Journal of Nonprofit & Public Sector Marketing.*

World Health Organization. 2005. *New Bangkok charter for health promotion adopted to address rapidly changing global health issue.* Retrieved from www.who.int/mediacentre/news/releases/2005/pr34/en/index.html.

World Health Organization. 2012. *The Ottawa charter for health promotion.* Retrieved from www.who.int/healthpromotion/conferences/previous/ottawa/en/index.html.

YMCA of Greater New York. 2011. *YMCA of Greater New York, financial statements 2010.* New York: YMCA of Greater New York.

INDEX

Note: The italicized *f* and *t* following page numbers refer to figures and tables, respectively.

A

accountability, in partnerships 33
Aconcagua expedition 97
ACT (AIDS Committee of Toronto) 125
activation, in corporate partnerships 30, 58
Active Healthy Kids Canada
overview of 24
The Partnership Protocol development and 23
performance monitoring in 173-174
Report Card on Physical Activity for Children and Youth 19
active transportation 15-16, 174, 177
AgênciaClick Isobar 42
agencies, in sponsorship 54
Agita São Paulo–Agita Mundo 136-137
AHL (American Hockey League) 142, 175
AIDS Committee of Toronto (ACT) 125
AIDS Walk for Life 124-125, 125*f*
alliances of nongovernmental organizations 34
ambush marketing 60
American Academy of Family Physicians 166*t*
American Alliance for Health, Physical Education, Recreation and Dance 158
American Association for Physical Activity and Recreation 158
American College of Sports Medicine 13
American Hockey League (AHL) 142, 175
American Society for Nutrition 13
antecedents of partnership 25
Arts for Children and Youth 139
ASC (Australian Sports Commission) 135

Ashoka Changemakers 140
association, in sponsorship 57-58
AstraZeneca Canada 139
athletes
as champions 102, 106, 112
in marketing programs 19, 52
negative public view of 175
as role models 94-98, 102
as targets of marketing 122-123
At My Best 139
Australian Sports Commission (ASC) 135

B

balance of power 26, 176
Bangkok Charter for Health Promotion in a Globalized World 179
behavioral change marketing 37, 37*t*
Belanger, Tammy 150-151, 151*f*
Bell Canada 92, 127
bias, in sponsored research 180-181
Bienenstock Natural Playgrounds 59
blogs 41
Boston College Center for Corporate Citizenship 81, 90
Boys and Girls Clubs
Canadian Tire Jumpstart Program and 20, 90
CATCH program and 157, 162, 163
Healthy Kids program and 139
branding
brand equity 8
in cause-related marketing 64, 90
partnership compatibility and 85-86

C

Cadbury 166*t*
Canada
corporate support in 76-77, 84, 90

fees for goods and services in 73
fitness levels in 14-15
foundation sources in 76
government funding sources in 71
philanthropic revenues in 73-74
sport and recreation organizations in 70-71
Canada Food Guide 39
Canada Games 145
Canada on the Move (COTM) initiative 37, 37*t*
Canada Post 127
Canadian AIDS Society 125
Canadian Association of Gift Planners 74
Canadian Breast Cancer Foundation 124, 124*f*
Canadian Centre for Ethics in Sport (CCES) 126-129
Canadian Diabetes Association (CDA) 147-149, 150-151
Canadian Directory to Foundations & Corporations 76
Canadian Heritage (PCH) 135
Canadian Imperial Bank of Commerce (CIBC) 53, 64, 124, 124*f*
Canadian Institutes of Health Research (CIHR) 27
Canadian Mental Health Association 31-32
Canadian Multicultural Hockey Championship 139
Canadian Partnership for Children's Health & Environment 139
Canadian Space Agency 20
Canadian Sponsorship Landscape Study (CSLS)
findings of 2
profile of a sponsee 65-66
profile of a sponsor 67
on size and scope of the sponsorship industry 57
on sponsorship evaluation 67

Canadian Sport Centre Atlantic 145

Canadian Team Sports Coalition 146

Canadian Tire Hockey School 120

Canadian Tire Jumpstart Program 20, 90

Canadian Women's Foundation 139

Cardio Cinema 43

CARE 141

CATCH (Coordinated Approach to Child Health) case study 154-164
  evidence from 156-157
  goals of 163
  Jared Foundation and 164
  overview of 154-155
  partnership components 158-159
  The Partnership Protocol and 159, 160*t*
  purpose of 161-162

category exclusivity 58, 60, 123

cause-related marketing 64, 90-91, 119

CCA (Concerned Children's Advertisers) 62-63, 89

CCES (Canadian Centre for Ethics in Sport) 126-129

CDA (Canadian Diabetes Association) 147-149, 150-151

CDC (U.S. Centers for Disease Control and Prevention) 137, 163

CDPAC (Chronic Disease Prevention Alliance of Canada) 34-36

celebrity presence 56, 148

Centre for Sport in Canadian Society management model 25-26

challenges to partnerships 175-181
  balance of power 26, 176
  competition from other organizations 176-177
  disconnect between partners and goals 32, 119, 120, 177
  food industry and 179
  internal communication 32-33
  management and 181-182
  sharing the burden of health promotion 180

champions
  athletes as 102, 104, 112
  celebrities as 56
  desirable characteristics of 105-106

functions of 98, 101-102, 129
  in ParticipACTION 107
  recruiting and retaining 107
  in Right To Play 106, 107
  role models and 94-98
  sport as a means of physical activity and 94

charitable gaming fees 73

charities. *See also* not-for-profit organizations; philanthropy
  celebrity presence 56
  donations 10
  image transfer in sponsorship 54-55
  importance of partnering with 55-57, 147-149

charity runs
  participant's perspective 150-151
  for raising awareness 146, 151
  Sudbury ROCKS!!! 147-149, 150-151

CHEO Research Institute 23*f*

children
  food marketing regulation and 35, 122
  obesity in 35-36

Children's Hospital of Eastern Ontario (CHEO) Research Institute 23*f*

Chronic Disease Prevention Alliance of Canada (CDPAC) 34-36

CIBC (Canadian Imperial Bank of Commerce) 53, 64, 124, 124*f*

CIHR (Canadian Institutes of Health Research) 27

cities. *See* municipalities

"clawback" clauses 174

Coalition for Adolescent Girls 140

Coca-Cola 166*t*

Coca-Cola Canada 8, 20, 59, 116-119

Cody-Cox, John-Paul 144-146, 144*f*

Cognitive Surplus—Creativity and Generosity in a Connected Age (Shirky) 48

collaboration
  in partnership continuum 11
  virtual 47

commercials, in sponsorships 58

Commonwealth Games Canada Partnership Filter and Application Toolkit 25

communications. *See also* marketing
  across cultures 44

champions and 98, 106
  external 33
  global connectedness 45-48
  importance of 31-32, 171, 172
  internal 32-33, 172
  prenegotiations 172
  public feedback 42
  strategies 32-33
  through social media 31, 41-42, 45-46
  web-based meetings 41

community awareness
  champions and 101-102, 106, 129
  sport and recreation facilities and 143, 146
  sport participation programs and 41
  strategies for 41
  virtual voice 48

Community Foundations of Canada 128

community partnerships
  with Canadian Diabetes Association 147
  charity runs 146, 151
  sport and recreation facilities 143, 146
  Sudbury ROCKS!!! 142, 147-149

competition from other organizations 176-177

Compton, Kevin 72, 98, 99-102, 99*f*

computers. *See also* social media
  Internet access 47
  in marketing 30
  as "tools of inactivity" 30-31, 43-44

Concerned Children's Advertisers (CCA) 62-63, 89

conflict of interest 180-181

conflict resolution 26, 64

Consensus Conference on Obesity 12-13

consumers, partnership benefits to 39

contracts, revenue from 72, 73

contributions, revenue from 72. *See also* donations

Coordinated Approach to Child Health. *See* CATCH (Coordinated Approach to Child Health) case study

Coordination Tool Kit 161

COPED model 171

corporate foundations 75, 86-87, 88, 140

corporate partnerships
  advice for managers on 64-65, 87, 100-101, 129

brand compatibility in 85-86, 126-127
return on investment in 63, 105, 123, 170
corporate social responsibility (CSR)
benefits to corporation 114-115
bringing other partners to the table 121
building own properties 119-120
examples of 124-125
image transfer and 53-54, 121
leveraging role models 120
profitability and 82-83
recognizing the cause 119
share value and 128-129
corporate sponsorship 52-68
activation in 58
association in 57-58
celebrity presence 56
commercials in 58
definition of 52-53
evaluation of 60
exclusivity in 58, 60, 123
finding not-for-profit sponsees for 66-67
finding sponsors for not-for-profits 60, 61t, 64-65
image transfer in 53-54, 121
as in-kind donations of goods and services 52, 88-89, 90, 124t
in the Olympic Games 52
in partnership continuum 9f, 10-11, 81
research bias and 180-181
size and scope of sponsorship industry 57
sponsee profiles 54, 65-66
sponsor profiles 67
stakeholders in 54
statistics on 76-77, 80, 84, 89, 90
strategic 57-58
corporate support 80-92
amounts of 82
benefits of 80
cause-related marketing 90-91, 119
donations 84, 88, 90
employee volunteering 91-92, 127
funding statistics 76-77, 80, 84
increasing demand for 81
industry type and 90
in-kind donations of goods and services 52, 88-89, 90, 124t
on partnership continuum 9-11, 9f, 81

reasons for 82-84, 83t
return on investment and 63, 105, 123, 170
risks in 85-88
types of support 81-82
COTM (Canada on the Move) initiative 37, 37t
Cranbrook Civic Arena Multiplex 143, 146
credibility, champions and 98
crisis management 26, 64
Crowdrise 42
crowd sourcing 42
CSLS. See Canadian Sponsorship Landscape Study
CSR. See corporate social responsibility
cultural diversity, communication and 44

D
Dallas Aerobic Institute 137
Day on Skates 120
decision making, balance of power and 176
Deeth, Bev 62-65, 62f
Dell Foundation 162
Dietitians of Canada 39
disconnect concept 32, 119, 120, 177
donations
corporate 84, 88
in-kind, of goods and services 52, 88-89, 90, 124t
motivation for 10
statistics on 73-74
Downsview Park 144-145
"Driving Partnerships With Quality and Credibility" (Hentges) 12-14

E
Eat Smart program 159
education sector
CATCH health-promotion study in 155-164
in partnerships for promotion 134-135
schools as program sites 9, 135
effectiveness
communication and planning and 172
COPED model of 171
factors in 171, 172t
leadership and 172-173
marketing plans and 30-31
measuring 170-171
The Partnership Protocol guidelines on 24-26
performance monitoring of 173-174
planning for setbacks 174-175

employee volunteering 91-92, 127
Esso Canada 8
ethnic diversity 44
evaluation
of partnerships 26, 173
of sponsorships 60
exclusivity, in corporate partnerships 58, 60, 123

F
facility funding
by municipalities 8, 15-16
by partnerships 8, 143, 146
FDA (Food and Drug Administration) 13
Federal Express (FedEx) 53
fees for goods and services 72-73
Fiat Brazil 42
FindingLife 66-67, 96-97
FindingLife (film) 96-97
Fire Prevention Canada 139
First Nation communities 108-111
FlagHouse, Inc. 157-159, 160t, 162-163
Flying Start 157
Food and Drug Administration (FDA) 13
food industry
marketing regulation of 13, 35, 122
nutritional labels 39
obesity and 35-36
research bias and 181
risks of partnerships with 178, 179
Forzani Group 139
Foundation Center 75-76
Foundation Directory Online 76
foundations
corporate 75, 86-87, 88, 140
grant-making 76
revenues from 75-76, 86-87
Framing Hope program 89

G
galas 87
gaming fees 73
Garnier FindingLife Expedition to Africa 66-67, 96-97
Gatorade 53, 122-123
Get Fit for Space With Dr. Bob Thirsk 20
"Get Inspired. Get Moving" campaign 19, 20
Giant Leap 157
Giant Tiger 128-129
Gifts in Kind International 89
Girls' Growth Fund IPO 139
Giving USA Foundation 76

Global Conference on Health Promotion, Thailand 179
Global Fund to Fight AIDS, Tuberculosis, and Malaria 102
global perspectives 135-138
  Agita São Paulo–Agita Mundo 136-137
  global commitment to health 179
  International Platform on Sport and Development 135-136, 140
  megaevents 137-138
  Nike and 140-141
  sharing the burden of health promotion 180
glossary of terms 209-212
goals
  disconnect between partners and 32, 119, 120, 177
  importance of clear 32
Going Strong 157
Good360 89
governments. *See also* municipalities
  challenging aspects of dealing with 72
  as funding sources 7-8, 71-72, 117, 117f, 145
  partnerships in advocacy roles to 35-36
  as seeking private sector funding 178-179
grant-making foundations 76
grants, government 72
GreenGym 20

H
HALO (Healthy Active Living and Obesity Research Group) 23, 24
Hamilton, Chuck 45-48, 45f
Hawaii Ironman Triathlon 53
health. *See also* obesity
  declines in 15
  global commitment to 179
  government spending cutbacks and 15
  marketing of unhealthy foods 35
Health Canada 39
health sector
  bias in partnerships 180-181
  partnership benefits for 14-16
  in partnerships for promotion 8, 134-135, 180
Healthy Active Living and Obesity Research Group (HALO) 23, 24
Healthy Kids 138-139

Healthy Kids, Healthy Schools 142
Hentges, Eric 12-14
Heritage Classic 120
hierarchical relationships 176
Hockey 101 139
Hockey Canada
  corporate donations of 84
  Forzani Group and 139
  Gatorade and 122
  partnerships of 8, 11, 85-86
Hockey Canada Foundation 86-87
Home Depot 89
Homeless World Cup 138
Houston, City of 142
HP Pavilion Management 100

I
IBM 166t
IBM Canada 164-165
IEG 57, 60
ILSI (International Life Sciences Institute) 12-14
image transfer 53-54, 121
Imagine Canada 76
Improve the Grade 19
inactivity crisis
  negative effects of 2, 14-15
  statistics on 43
  using tools of inactivity to promote physical activity 30-31, 43-44
infrastructure funding 72
in-kind donations of goods and services
  examples of 88, 124t
  recipients of 90
  software 89
  in sponsorships 52
  through intermediaries 89
Inspire the Nation 1
Intact Insurance 120
internal communication, partnership 32-33
International Life Sciences Institute (ILSI) 12-14
International Olympic Committee 138, 177
International Platform on Sport and Development 135-136, 140
International Sport and Culture Association (ISCA) 135
International Union for Health Promotion and Education (IUHPE) 137
Internet 47. *See also* computers; social media
investment, in corporate sponsorship 58

Investors Group 127-128
ISCA (International Sport and Culture Association) 135
IUHPE (International Union for Health Promotion and Education) 137

J
Jared Foundation 159, 163
Jewish General Hospital 125

K
Kellogg Canada 37, 38-40, 40f, 166t
Kellogg Nutrition Symposium (KNS) 39
Kicking AIDS Out 136
Kids Help Phone 139
Kieran Pathways Society 177
Kings Care Foundation 56
Kraft Foods 166t

L
Larsen, Craig 34-36, 34f
Laureus Sport for Good Foundation 135
leadership in partnerships 172-173
Learn to Camp at Ontario Parks 43-44
Leyton Orient Community Sports Programme 142, 166t
life-streaming sites. *See* social media
linkage models 9-11, 9f
Logan, Aaron 55-57, 55f
Lowry, Christine 38-40, 40f
Lusk, Steve 161-164

M
MAA (Ministry of Aboriginal Affairs) 109, 112
Maasai Wilderness Conservation Trust (MWCT) 106
MacDonald, Lauren K. 122-123
MacKinnon, Jennifer 147-149
Mak, Camon 103-105, 103f
management of partnerships, model for 25-26
managers of not-for-profit organizations, advice for 64-65, 87, 100-101, 129
marketing. *See also* communications; corporate sponsorship
  across cultures 44
  ambush 60
  for behavioral change 37, 37t
  cause-related 64, 90-91, 119
  disconnect between partners and 32, 119, 120, 177
  internal communication and 30

promoting health and wellness 40

social media and 30, 31, 41-42

sponsorship as 52-53

"tools of inactivity" in 30-31, 43-44

of unhealthy foods and beverages 35-36

using sport in 31-32

marketing plans 30-31

market research agencies 54

Mars Inc. 166*t*

Mathare Youth Sports Association (MYSA) 141

McConnell Foundation 75, 127-128

media. *See also* social media

as advocates for physical activity 9

in partnerships 9, 63, 135

providing airtime 63

megaevents 137-138

megasponsees 65

Melia, Paul 126-129, 126*f*

membership fees 72

MEND (Mind, Exercise, Nutrition, Do-It) 163

messaging. *See also* communications; marketing

brand equity 8

in cause-related marketing 64, 90-91, 119

consistency in 40

partnership guidelines and 85-86

micro-philanthropy partnerships 8

Mike Weir Foundation 10, 102

Ministry of Aboriginal Affairs (MAA) 109, 112

monitoring of partnership performance 173-174

Montreal, City of 87

Montreal Canadiens Hockey Club 87

Moose Cree First Nation 108

Moran, Dave 115, 116-119, 116*f*

Moss Park Rejuvenation project 59

motivation

for corporate support 82-84, 83*t*

for *The Partnership Protocol* development 23

from partnerships 62

for philanthropy 74

Mount Kenya Expedition 97

Multicultural Markets 103-105

Multiplex 146

municipalities

active transportation options in 16

community awareness strategies of 41

corporate grants to 104

in partnerships 16, 87, 100

as revenue sources 71

mutual respect, in partnerships 63-64

MWCT (Maasai Wilderness Conservation Trust) 106

MYSA (Mathare Youth Sports Association) 141

N

National Association for Sport and Physical Education 158

National Center for Genome Research 166*t*

National Dairy Council 142

National Hockey League 72, 120

national perspectives 138-139, 142

national product creation 139, 142

NCDO (Dutch National Committee for International Cooperation and Sustainable Development) 135

netnography 31

Network of Provincial and Territorial Alliances 34

NGOs. *See* nongovernmental organizations

NIF (Norwegian Olympic and Paralympic Committee and Confederation of Sports) 135

Nike 135, 140-141

NikeCARE 141

Nike Changemakers 140-141

Nike Foundation 140

Nike Gamechangers 141

nongovernmental organizations (NGOs). *See also* not-for-profit organizations

alliances of 34-35

funding for 117, 118

Norwegian Olympic and Paralympic Committee and Confederation of Sports (NIF) 135

not-for-profit organizations

activation in corporate partnerships 58

advice for seeking corporate partnerships 64-65, 87, 100-101, 129

association in corporate partnerships 57-58, 85-86, 87

building owned properties 119-120

cause associated with 64, 90-91, 119

compatibility with corporate relationships 85-86, 126-127

corporate employee volunteering and 91-92, 127

disconnect between partners and goals 32, 119, 120, 177

distrust of for-profit organizations in 175

donations to 73-75

exclusivity in corporate partnerships 58, 60, 123

finding sponsors for 60, 61*t*, 64-65

funding trends for 2

government funding of 7-8, 71-72, 117, 117*f*, 145

image transfer in sponsorships 53-54

relationship building by 63

revenue strategies for 70-77, 80-81

small organizations 81

social media and 42

sponsee profile 65-66

sport and recreation organizations 70-71, 73, 75, 84, 90

value of corporate support of 85

nutritional labels on food 39

Nutrition Extension Programs 13

O

obesity

childhood 35-36

consensus conference on 12-13

food and beverage marketing and 35-36

inactivity crisis and 2, 14-15, 43-44

Olympic Games

global perspectives of 137-138

sponsorship in 52, 60, 67

online systems for partnerships 33

Ontario Ministry of Health Promotion 178-180

Ottawa Charter for Health Promotion 178

Ottawa, City of 8

Ottawa Superdome Sports Centre 8

Outrunning Cancer 42

P

Pan American Games 52, 144-145

Parent's Jury program (Australia) 36

Parks Canada 59
ParticipACTION. *See also The
    Partnership Protocol*
  Canadian Tire Jumpstart
    Program 20, 90
  champions in 107
  Coca-Cola Canada partner-
    ship 8, 59, 118
  Get Fit for Space With Dr.
    Bob Thirsk 20
  "Get Inspired. Get Moving"
    campaign 19
  GreenGym 20
  Improve the Grade 19
  on the inactivity crisis 15
  Inspire the Nation 20
  Moss Park Rejuvenation
    project 59
  operations of 19
  in *The Partnership Protocol*
    development 18, 21-24
  Sogo Active 20, 41, 126
  specific initiatives of 19-20
  Speed Skating Canada 145
partnership continuum 9-11,
    9*f*, 81
Partnership Filter and Applica-
    tion 25
Partnership for Philanthropic
    Planning 74
The Partnership Protocol 18-26
  CATCH and 159, 160*t*, 161
  development of 18-19, 22-24,
    22*f*
  motivation behind 23
  overview of 21, 21*f*
  on partner disconnect 58, 119,
    120, 177
  partnership guidelines in
    24-26
  science behind developing
    185-187
  text of 189-203
partnerships, public–private
  across sectors 8-9, 134-135
  benefits of 8, 11, 12, 15-16,
    63
  building and maintaining
    56-57
  challenges to 175-181
  collaborative 11, 47
  community perspectives on
    142-143, 146, 151
  on a continuum 9-11, 9*f*, 81
  crisis management in 26, 64
  definition of 6-7
  donation increases with 75
  effectiveness of 24-26, 30-31,
    170-173, 172*t*
  employee volunteering in
    91-92, 127

examples of 7-8
  with First Nation communi-
    ties 108-111
  future of 118
  global perspectives 135-138,
    140-141, 179-180
  importance of selecting the right
    partner 25, 117-118
  key learnings from 166*t*-167*t*
  management of 181-182
  messaging and 40-42, 64,
    85-86, 90-91, 110
  mutual respect in 63-64
  national perspectives 138-
    139, 142
  need for 1-3, 7-8
  objectives gap in 2-3
  performance monitoring of
    173-174
  planning for setbacks 174-175
  private partners in 1-3, 7-8,
    11, 108-109
  public–private, definition 7-8
  role of 14-16
  stakeholders in 32, 54, 116,
    117*f*
  "sweet spot" in 40, 40*f*
  trust in 36
  types of partners in 108-109
PCH (Canadian Heritage) 135
pedometers, distribution of 37
PepsiCo 122, 166*t*
Perdue, Vince 147-149
performance monitoring, in
    partnerships 173-174
performance requirements 174
personal relationships 181-182
philanthropy. *See also* charities;
    corporate support
  donations 73-74, 90
  foundations 75-76, 86-87
  motivation for 74
  in partnership continuum 10,
    81
physical activity
  active transportation 15-16,
    174, 177
  in disadvantaged youth 44
  government spending cutbacks
    and 15
  health benefits of 14-15
  Improve the Grade 19
  inactivity crisis 2, 14-15, 43-44
  partnership benefits for 14-16
  using social media to promote
    43-44
  using tools of inactivity to
    encourage 30-31, 43-44
Physical Activity Network of
    the Americas (RAFA-
    PANA) 137

Physical and Health Education
    Canada 139
planning for setbacks 174-175
PLAY (Promoting Life-Skills in
    Aboriginal Youth) 108-111
Play Hockey 104
podcasts 41
Positive Living Society of British
    Columbia 125
PPP. *See* partnerships, public–
    private
prenegotiations 172
President's Council on Physical
    Fitness and Sport 166*t*
Princess Margaret Hospital
    Foundation 125
private partners
  benefits of public partners 8
  collaboration with 11
  examples of 7-8
  philanthropy of 10
  sponsorship by 10-11
Project Adventure 157
Promoting Life-Skills in Aborig-
    inal Youth (PLAY) 108-111
public feedback 42
public–private partnerships
    (PPP). *See* partnerships,
    public–private
public sector, examples of 7-8

R
RAFA-PANA (Physical Activity
    Network of the Americas)
    137
RBC. *See* Royal Bank of Canada
recognition, champions and 98
*Report Card on Physical Activity
    for Children and Youth*
    (Active Healthy Kids
    Canada) 19
research
  "second harvest" from 13-14
  social media and 31
  sponsored 180-181
responsiveness, in partnerships
    173-174
return on investment (ROI) 63,
    105, 123, 170
revenues 70-77. *See also* corpo-
    rate support
  dependency on one funder
    for 88
  donations 10, 73-74, 84, 88, 90
  fees for goods and services
    72-73
  forms of 71-72
  from foundations 75-76, 86-87
  government sources of 7-8,
    71-72, 117, 117*f*, 145
  infrastructure funding 72

of sport and recreation organizations 70-71
statistics on 70
tactics to attract nonfinancial resources 123, 124*t*
Right To Play (RTP)
athlete ambassadors and 106
champions in 107-112
global perspectives of 31, 136
Nike partnership with 140
overview of 108, 136
partnership with First Nation communities 108-111, 112
risks in partnerships. *See* challenges to partnerships
Road Hockey to Conquer Cancer 55
Roadrunner partnership 175
ROI (return on investment) 63, 105, 123, 170
role models 94-98
athletes as 94-98, 102
attracting resources with 124*t*
champions and 98
composition of 94-95, 98
definition of 94
leveraging 120
recruitment of 124*t*
Roll Back Malaria Partnership 102
Royal Bank of Canada (RBC)
Canadian Open 10
funding statistics of 81
return on investment for 105
Wicket Cricket 103-104
Royal Bank of Canada Foundation 75, 81, 105
RTP. *See* Right To Play
Run for the Cure (CIBC) 53, 64, 124, 124*f*
Runner's World 42

S
Safe Kids Canada 138-139
Salmon, Art 178-180, 179*f*
Sandy Lake First Nation 108
San Jose, City of 100
San Jose Sharks 72, 100, 101
Save the Children 166*t*
School Physical Activity and Nutrition (SPAN) study 157
schools
CATCH health-promotion study in 155-164
in partnerships 9
as program sites 9, 135
scientific integrity, sponsorships and 181
SCORE Sports Coaches' Outreach programs 136

Scotiabank 124-125
screen time, physical activity and 43-44
SDC (Swiss Agency for Development and Cooperation) 135
"second harvest" concept 13-14
setbacks, planning for 174-175
share value/share capital 128-129
Shoppers Drug Mart 125, 125*f*
Silicon Valley Sports & Entertainment 100
Smith, Scott 84, 85-88, 85*f*
social media
attracting nonfinancial resources for activation 124*t*
communicating through 31, 41-42, 45-46
crowd sourcing in 42
Internet access and 47
level playing field on 48
in messaging and marketing 30, 31, 41-42
promoting physical activity through 43-44
public feedback in 42
as source of secondary research 31
sweeping changes from 45-48
social networking sites. *See* social media
social news-sharing sites 41. *See also* social media
SOCOG (Sydney Organising Committee for the Olympic Games) 138
software companies 89
Sogo Active
goals of 20
partnership with Coca-Cola 126
use of social media 41
SPAN (School Physical Activity and Nutrition) study 157
Spark Together for Healthy Kids 139
Special Olympics Canada 158
Special Olympics USA 158
Speed Skating Canada 120, 145
sponsees 54, 65-66
sponsorship. *See* corporate sponsorship
sport
as corporate marketing tool 31-32
health benefits of 14
inactivity crisis and 14-15
public view of 175

Sport and Development Partnership Toolkit 136
sport and recreation organizations
corporate support of 84, 90
definition of 70
foundation support of 75
revenue data on 70-71, 73
sponsorship of 90
Sport Canada 145
Sport for a Better World 140-141
Sport for Social Change Network (SSCN) 141
sport sector 134-135
SSCN (Sport for Social Change Network) 141
stakeholders
framework to engage 32
groups in 54, 116, 117*f*
Steve Nash Foundation 102
Sudbury ROCKS!!! 147-149, 150-151
Sumitomo Chemical 102
Sun Life Financial 20
supplements 126, 181
Swiss Agency for Development and Cooperation (SDC) 135
Sydney Organising Committee for the Olympic Games (SOCOG) 138

T
Team Up Foundation 56
technology
to encourage physical activity 37, 43-44
as "tools of inactivity" 30-31, 43-44
TechSoup Global 89
Tennis Canada 33, 173
ThinkFirst program 139, 142
Thunderbird Management 8
Today's Parent 138
Toronto, City of 142, 175
Toronto Community Housing 59
Toronto Maple Leafs 56
transparency, need for 33
Tremblay, Mark 22-24, 22*f*
True Sport 75, 127-128
trust, importance of 36
Twitter 46-47

U
UEFA (Union of European Football Associations) 135
UNICEF Canada 166*t*
Union of European Football Associations (UEFA) 135
unique selling properties (USPs) 64

United National Inter-Agency
Taskforce on Sport for
Development and Peace 14
United Nations Foundation 140
United States
  corporate support in 76,
    84, 90
  dietary guidelines of 39
  fees for goods and services
    in 73
  foundation funding sources
    in 75-76
  government funding sources
    in 71-72
  philanthropic revenues in 73
  sport and recreation organi-
    zations in 70
United States Department of
  Agriculture (USDA) 166t
United States Olympic Committee (USOC) 52
universities, in partnerships
  164-165, 166t-167t

University of Texas 142, 157-
  159, 160t, 161-163
U.S. Centers for Disease Con-
  trol and Prevention (CDC)
  137, 163
USAID 166t
USOC (United States Olympic
  Committee) 52
USPs (unique selling properties)
  64

V
Vancouver Organizing Committee 176-177
virtual collaborators 47
Volleyball Canada 144-145

W
Waters Corporation 166t
websites 41-42, 44, 47
Weekend to End Women's Cancers 125, 125f
WHO (World Health Organization) 137, 179

Wicket Cricket 103-104
Wilson Sporting Goods 20, 90
women, empowerment of 101
World Aquatics Championships
  114
World Bank 166t
World Health Organization
  (WHO) 137, 179
World Wildlife Fund 116

Y
YMCA
  CATCH and 162, 163
  FlagHouse and 157
  Healthy Kids program and 139
  revenues of 70
  as sport and recreation organi-
    zation 71
  Strong Kids 1K 148, 149

ABOUT THE AUTHORS

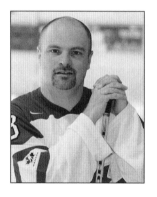

Norman O'Reilly, PhD, is a professor with the University of Ottawa's faculty of health sciences, specializing in sport business. He was recently named a lifetime research fellow of the North American Society for Sport Management and was the 2011 recipient of the University of Ottawa's Media Excellence Award. He is also a senior advisor with TrojanOne, a Toronto-based marketing agency, where he works with corporations and properties on revenue generation and sponsorship. O'Reilly holds a PhD in management from the Sprott School of Business at Carleton University, an MBA from the Telfer School of Management at the University of Ottawa, an MA in sports administration from the University of Ottawa, and a BSc in kinesiology from the University of Waterloo.

O'Reilly is an active researcher and has published 5 books, more than 50 articles in refereed management journals, and more than 100 conference proceedings and case studies in the areas of sport management, sponsorship, tourism marketing, risk management, sport finance, and social marketing. Dr. O'Reilly is the lead researcher on the Canadian Sponsorship Landscape Study, a highlight of the annual Canadian Sponsorship Forum since 2007, currently in its sixth edition.

O'Reilly competes in triathlons, long-distance runs, cross-country skiing events, and ice hockey leagues and tournaments. He has completed six Ironman triathlons and represented Canada at five long-distance World Triathlon Championships in his age group, finishing as high as 17th in 1997. He is an active mountain climber and an avid world traveler, having visited more than 40 countries.

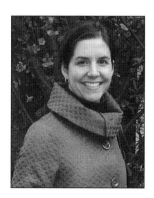

Michelle Brunette, MHK, teaches international health in the School of Human Kinetics and is an academic advisor at Laurentian University in Ontario, Canada. She received her master of human kinetics from Laurentian University, a BA in political science from the University of Windsor, and an honors bachelor of physical and health education from Laurentian University.

Brunette has published in the *Journal of Sport Behavior* and has presented at several conferences.

She is a volunteer coordinator for the Sudbury Rocks!!! Race, Run or Walk for Diabetes, a founding board executive for the Young Professionals Association, and the former athlete representative for Ringette Ontario. She has extensive cross-cultural work experience: She taught conversational English and Canadian culture to students in China, served as a TESL instructor preparing people for teaching and working abroad, and worked in Ireland as part of the Student Work Abroad program. She is a keen explorer who has worked or traveled in more than 20 countries.

Brunette is an avid runner, participating in both marathons and half marathons. She also enjoys hiking, canoeing, and playing soccer. When not working, Brunette enjoys spending time with her favorite partners: husband Jamie, daughters Malin and Nellie, and golden retreiver Charlie.